NLN CORE COMPETENCIES FOR NURSE EDUCATORS
A DECADE OF INFLUENCE

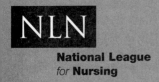

National League
for **Nursing**

NLN CORE COMPETENCIES FOR NURSE EDUCATORS

A DECADE OF INFLUENCE

Edited by:

Judith A. Halstead, PhD, RN, ANEF, FAAN

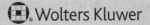

. Wolters Kluwer

Philadelphia · Baltimore · New York · London
Buenos Aires · Hong Kong · Sydney · Tokyo

Vice President and Publisher: Julie K. Stegman
Executive Editor: Kelley Squazzo
Director of Product Development: Jennifer K. Forestieri
Senior Development Editor: Meredith L. Brittain
Marketing Manager: Katie Schlesinger
Editorial Assistant: Leo Gray
Design Coordinator: Steven Druding
Production Project Manager: Joan Sinclair
Manufacturing Coordinator: Karin Duffield
Prepress Vendor: Aptara, Inc.

Halstead, J. A. (2019). *NLN Core Competencies for Nurse Educators: A Decade of Influence.* Washington, DC: National League for Nursing.

Library of Congress Cataloging-in-Publication Data

Names: Halstead, Judith A., editor. | National League for Nursing, issuing
  body.
Title: NLN core competencies for nurse educators : a decade of influence /
  edited by Judith Halstead.
Other titles: National League for Nursing core competencies for nurse
  educators
Description: Washington, D.C. : NLN, National League for Nursing;
  Philadelphia : Wolters Kluwer, [2019] | Includes bibliographical
  references.
Identifiers: LCCN 2018032865 | ISBN 9781975104276
Subjects: | MESH: Faculty, Nursing—standards | Clinical
  Competence—standards | Education, Nursing—standards | Nurse's Role |
  Review
Classification: LCC RT71 | NLM WY 19.1 | DDC 610.73071/1—dc23
LC record available at https://lccn.loc.gov/2018032865

DRC0818

About the Editor

Judith A. Halstead, PhD, RN, ANEF, FAAN is Executive Director of the National League for Nursing Commission for Nursing Education Accreditation in Washington, DC, a position she has held since July 2014. She has over 35 years of experience in nursing education, with expertise in online education, nurse educator competencies, and evidence-based teaching in nursing education. She is coeditor of the widely referenced book on nursing education, *Teaching in Nursing: A Guide for Faculty.* Dr. Halstead is the recipient of numerous awards including the MNRS Advancement of Science Award for the Nursing Education Research Section and the Sigma Theta Tau International Elizabeth Russell Belford Excellence in 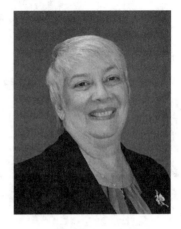 Education Award. She is a fellow in the NLN Academy of Nursing Education and the American Academy of Nursing. She served as the president of the National League for Nursing from 2011 to 2013.

About the Contributors

Linda Caputi, EdD, RN, CNE, ANEF is Professor Emeritus, College of DuPage. She has taught in LPN, ADN, BSN, and MSN programs. She is President of Linda Caputi Inc., a nursing education consulting company. Dr. Caputi has consulted with hundreds of schools for over 30 years on topics related to revising curriculum, teaching students to think, developing a concept-based curriculum, transforming clinical education, test item writing and analysis, using an evidence-based model for NCLEX success, and numerous other nursing education topics. She has also presented at hundreds of workshops and nursing education conferences. She has published journal articles, educational software programs, and books, the most recent being the student textbook *Think Like a Nurse: A Handbook*. Dr. Caputi is a Certified Nurse Educator, was inducted as a fellow into NLN's Academy of Nursing Education, has served on the NLN's Board of Governors, and is a site visitor for the NLN's Commission for Nursing Education Accreditation.

Linda S. Christensen, EdD, JD, RN, CNE is currently the chief governance officer for the National League for Nursing in Washington, DC. She previously was the chief administration officer at the National League for Nursing, a position she held from 2009 through 2017. She has more than 35 years of experience in nursing education, with expertise in nursing educator competencies, nursing education, curriculum, and evaluation. She has taught both graduate and undergraduate nursing, as well as online education courses. Additionally, she is an attorney with 20 years' experience of combining nursing and the law. She is frequently a guest speaker on legal issues in nursing education and has authored chapters on nursing law for various books on nursing education.

Kristina Thomas Dreifuerst, PhD, RN, CNE, ANEF is an Associate Professor in the College of Nursing at Marquette University in Milwaukee, Wisconsin. She has been a nurse educator for the past 22 years and has focused her expertise in faculty development, curriculum development, and evaluation on preparing nurses for faculty roles. Her research is at the forefront of disciplinary efforts to (1) develop, use, and test innovative teaching methods to improve students' clinical reasoning skills and (2) investigate how teachers can best be prepared to use evidence-based teaching and learning methods. Dr. Dreifuerst is the recipient of numerous national and international awards recognizing the contribution of her research to the field. She has been credentialed as a Certified Nurse Educator since 2009.

Alecia Schneider Fox, PhD, APRN, FNP-BC is an assistant professor at Drexel University in Philadelphia, Pennsylvania, where she has taught in the BSN and MSN programs for 12 years. Her clinical experience consists of advanced practice nursing in emergency and trauma. Dr. Fox also has expertise in faculty development and leadership. Her research activity has examined the experience of nurse faculty new to a full-time academic role and their intent to stay in academia.

Betsy Frank, PhD, RN, ANEF is Professor Emerita at Indiana State University. She also serves as Associate Director of Accreditation for the National League for Nursing Commission for Nursing Education Accreditation (NLN-CNEA). She has over 40 years of teaching experience, most recently in an online RN-BSN program at Indiana State University. She has been active in the NLN including as chair of several councils. Dr. Frank has published many articles and book chapters on topics pertinent to nursing education. In 2011, she received the National League for Nursing's Excellence in Teaching Award and she was in the initial cadre of Academy of Nurse Educator Fellows.

Marilyn Frenn, PhD, RN, CNE, FTOS, ANEF, FAAN is professor and director of the PhD program at Marquette University, Milwaukee, Wisconsin. She teaches the PhD nursing education research, policy, and leadership course, as well as the graduate nursing research and evidence for practice course, the graduate health promotion course, and the undergraduate culture and health course. She helped to get interprofessional education (IPE) initiatives started at Marquette University in collaboration with the Medical College of Wisconsin and currently serves as the Nursing IPE Liaison. She is active in the National League for Nursing, where she currently serves as a member of the Commission for Nursing Education Accreditation Standards Committee. She has previously served on the Membership Committee, on the Board of Governors, and as President of the Wisconsin League for Nursing. She previously served on the CNE Certification Commission and as chair of the CNE Test Development Committee and several CNE exam item-writing teams. She has published and presented in the areas of teaching excellence preparing for the Certified Nurse Educator (CNE) examination and of IPE. Dr. Frenn is credentialed as a certified nurse educator and is a fellow in the Academy of Nursing Education, the Obesity Society, and the American Academy of Nursing.

Dawn M. Gordon, PhD, MS, MBA, RN, PHN is the Dean of Nursing and Sciences at Minnesota West Community and Technical College in Worthington, Minnesota, where she has directed ADN and PN programs for 13 years. Dr. Gordon has served in nursing education, leadership, and administration in rural and underserved communities for 18 years. Her clinical experience consists of cardiac care/critical care, medical/surgical, and emergency nursing. Dr. Gordon researches nursing leadership successes and educational learning strategies (such as collaborative testing) in the rural community. Dr. Gordon received her doctorate of philosophy (PhD) from South Dakota State University, her master's of management and master's of business administration (MBA) from Colorado Technical University, and a bachelor of arts in nursing from Augustana University. She is cochair of the ADN/PN Program Deans and Directors leadership group in Minnesota. Dr. Gordon currently serves as vice president of a rural hospital advisory board.

Jennifer Hedrick-Erickson, MSN, RN, CNL is an Associate Professor and BSN Completion Program Coordinator at Viterbo University, in La Crosse, Wisconsin. She has taught in the completion program for 18 years, and coordinated the program for 10 years. She has held a number of leadership roles at the university, in program review among others. Her clinical experience consists of medical/surgical nursing, obstetrics, and emergency nursing. Jennifer has expertise in curriculum development and online teaching, specializing in andragogy. Her scholarship focused on using hermeneutics and phenomenology in student nursing education and patient education for those residing in rural settings. She is a member of the Wisconsin Nurses and American Nurses Association and Sigma Theta Tau International Honor Society of Nursing.

Anne M. Krouse, PhD, MBA, RN-BC is professor and Dean of the School of Nursing at Widener University. Her clinical experience is in the areas of maternal-child health and she is certified in Nursing Informatics. Dr. Krouse has 19 years of expertise as a faculty member, teaching in undergraduate, master's, DNP, and PhD nursing programs. Her areas of research include leadership development in nurse faculty, active learning, and self-directed learning. Dr. Krouse is active in the National League for Nursing, where she currently serves as Treasurer and a member of the Board of Governors. She previously served as a member of the Public Policy Committee.

Susan Luparell, PhD, RN, CNE, ANEF is an Associate Professor in the College of Nursing at Montana State University, Bozeman, Montana, where she has been involved in both the baccalaureate and graduate nursing programs for 20 years. A fellow in the Academy of Nursing Education, Susan is an expert on the dynamics between teacher and learner in nursing education, as well as a nationally recognized speaker and author on the topic of incivility in nursing education. Her scholarship focuses on the ethical implications of incivility in health care, including how it affects others and how it can be managed in academic and in clinical settings. Additionally, Susan is a seasoned instructor who has received multiple commendations over the years for excellence in teaching.

Bette Mariani, PhD, RN, ANEF is an Associate Professor of Nursing at Villanova University M. Louise Fitzpatrick College of Nursing and a Fellow in the NLN Academy of Nursing Education. She is President of the International Nursing Association for Clinical Simulation and Learning (INACSL), and is recognized as a leader for her contributions in nursing education and simulation. Her work, which focuses on improving the quality and rigor of simulation, adds breadth and depth to the science of nursing education. She is dedicated to advancing the science of nursing education through research and scholarship addressing educational strategies, assessment, evaluation, and instrument development. She has worked tirelessly with students and colleagues to move the agenda of nursing education research forward through the dissemination of multiple papers and presentations. This work, as well as her involvement in INACSL and the NLN, continues to lead to significant changes in the quality of simulation and nursing education.

Kristen McLaughlin, MSN, RN, CPNP-PC is an assistant clinical professor at Drexel University in Philadelphia, Pennsylvania, where she has taught in the BSN program for six years. She is a doctoral student at Widener University, currently in the dissertation stage. Her research interest is in the doctoral preparation of academic nurse educators. She is credentialed as a pediatric nurse practitioner. Her clinical experience is in pediatrics with clinical expertise in pediatric orthopedics and sports medicine.

Barbara J. Patterson, PhD, RN, ANEF is a Distinguished Professor and Director of the PhD Program in the School of Nursing and Associate Dean for Scholarship and Inquiry at Widener University in Chester, Pennsylvania. She is also the Distinguished Scholar in the NLN/Chamberlain Center for Advancing the Science of Nursing Education. She received her PhD from the University of Rhode Island. She teaches doctoral students qualitative research, nursing science/theory, leadership, and dissertation advisement. She has chaired over 45 PhD dissertations, many investigating nursing education topics. Dr. Patterson has presented and published extensively in nursing education, specifically in the areas of evidence-based teaching, veterans' transitions, and leadership in nursing education. She was a faculty member for the Nurse Faculty Leadership Academy of Sigma Theta Tau International (STTI) working with novice nurse educators and leadership development. Dr. Patterson was Chair of NLN's Research Review Panel from 2012 to 2015, which reviews nursing education research grants. Dr. Patterson is the Research Briefs Editor for *Nursing Education Perspectives*.

Martha M. Scheckel, PhD, RN is Dean and Professor in the College of Nursing, Health, and Human Behavior at Viterbo University in La Crosse, Wisconsin. She has 14 years of academic experience, teaching in undergraduate and graduate nursing programs. She was instrumental in laying the groundwork for the first edition of the *Nurse Educator Competencies: Creating an Evidence-Based Practice for Nurse Educators* when she was a doctoral student at the University of Wisconsin-Madison's School of Nursing. Her publications have centered on using phenomenology and hermeneutics to study nursing and patient education. She has expertise in curriculum design and development and academic leadership. She has authored a chapter in Diane Billings and Judith Halstead's *Teaching in Nursing: A Guide for Faculty*; was a mentor for the Sigma Theta Tau International Honor Society of Nursing, Nurse Faculty Leadership Academy; and is a Fellow in the Leadership for Academic Nursing Program through the American Association of Colleges of Nursing.

Jennifer A. Specht, PhD, RN is the Founding Director of the Department of Nursing, Cabrini University in Radnor, Pennsylvania. Her clinical experience consists of postsurgical and cardiothoracic intensive care nursing. Dr. Specht has expertise in mentoring and faculty development, curriculum development and evaluation, and leadership. She served on the Board of Directors for the Mu Omicron Chapter of Sigma Theta Tau at DeSales University, and has reviewed grant funding proposals related to her areas of expertise. Her research interests include mentoring, leadership, and social justice; she also codeveloped the Model of New Normal focused on addressing parents' experiences related to their chronically ill children. She has authored chapters in medical-surgical and research textbooks. Dr. Specht has published and presented her work nationally and internationally.

Darrell Spurlock Jr., PhD, RN, NEA-BC, ANEF is an Associate Professor of Nursing and Director of the Leadership Center for Nursing Education Research at Widener University in Chester, Pennsylvania. As a nurse-academic psychologist, Dr. Spurlock has published and presented widely in the areas of educational research methodology, measurement, assessment, statistical analysis, and evidence-based practice (EBP). In addition to teaching responsibilities in the PhD and DNP programs at Widener University, Dr. Spurlock is a principal investigator or coinvestigator on studies examining the clinical education experiences of family nurse practitioner students, nurses' and nursing students' EBP knowledge and attitudes, and several methodology-related subjects. Dr. Spurlock is a member of the NLN Commission for Nursing Education Accreditation (CNEA) Program Review Committee and is a frequent workshop presenter and quantitative methods consultant. In 2016 he became the inaugural editor of the *Journal of Nursing Education* (*JNE*) Methodology Corner column. Dr. Spurlock currently serves as Assistant Editor of *JNE*.

Theresa M. "Terry" Valiga, EdD, RN, CNE, ANEF, FAAN is Professor Emerita at the Duke University School of Nursing, a Fellow for the PhD program at the Villanova University College of Nursing, and Senior Visiting Professor at the Virginia Commonwealth University School of Nursing. She holds a BS from Trenton State College and an MEd and EdD, both in Nursing Education, from Teachers College, Columbia University. She held faculty appointments at Duke, Trenton State, Seton Hall, Georgetown, Villanova, and Fairfield (where she served as dean), and she served as the NLN's Chief Program Officer for nine years during which time book publications were revitalized and several signature programs were launched including certification for nurse educators, the Centers of Excellence in Nursing Education, and the Academy of Nurse Educators. Dr. Valiga has published extensively, received grants to support education-focused research, received all major national awards in education, and provided leadership in the field through writing, speaking, consulting, teaching, and mentoring.

Foreword

In the 13 years since the Core Competencies of Nurse Educators were identified by a task group of the National League for Nursing, the evidence from which the core competencies and task statements were derived has revolutionized the landscape of nursing education. There was a surge of nurse educator preparation focus areas added to master's, post-master's, and doctoral programs based on the nurse educator competencies. The competencies formed the framework, supported by two job analyses, for a certification exam; currently, more than 6,100 faculty hold the coveted credential. Using the competency framework, faculty have developed assessment tools to identify student and faculty knowledge about the faculty role. Evidence-based educational practices dominate teaching and learning in the classroom, resource centers, and clinical practice sites. Using the evidence from the first edition, faculty have added to the science of nursing education to lead changes in practice and policy nationally and globally.

Inspired by the outcomes of the first edition, the National League for Nursing has once again assembled a panel of experts to synthesize current evidence for best practices in nursing education. This edition, while retaining the original framework for nurse educator competencies, provides the blueprint for implementing the role of the nurse educator into the future. In each chapter, readers will find thoughtful reviews of the evidence for each competency gleaned from research from 2005 to 2017.

The book concludes with a synthesis of the cross-competency findings, identification of gaps in the literature, and a guide to the next steps that will continue to define the evolving role of the nurse educator. The findings are discussed in the context of current recommendations for radical change in preparing health care professionals to meet future health care needs, and advocates for the role of the nurse educator as a part of system change. Faculty, students, and researchers will find not only a conceptual framework for educator preparation and role development but also a framework for programs of research that more closely link the role of the nurse educator as a driving force for improving patient care. Nurse educators, grounded by the current evidence about the role of the nurse educator, will ensure that the next generation of students is prepared to provide interdisciplinary, patient-focused, safe, and high-quality care.

Diane M. Billings, EdD, RN, ANEF, FAAN
Chancellor's Professor Emeritus
Indiana University School of Nursing, Indianapolis

Preface

This book reflects the second review of literature related to the NLN Core Competencies of Nurse Educators and underscores the influence the core competencies have had on the role of the academic nurse educator since they were first published in 2005. Throughout the United States and with increasing international influence, the educator competencies are being used to guide the development of graduate nursing programs designed to prepare future nursing faculty, define the roles and responsibilities of the nurse educator role, and provide a framework for the design of research studies to further explicate the knowledge, skills, and attitudes nurse educators need to effectively embrace the role. The core competencies also serve as the framework for the test blueprint of the NLN nurse educator certification examination. Since the establishment of the certification examination, over 6,000 nurse educators as of this printing have achieved certification as a nurse educator.

Chapter 1 briefly describes the process used by the original task group to conduct the first literature review from which the core competencies and their task statements were formulated, as well as the influence the core competencies have had on nursing education over the past 13 years. Chapter 2 summarizes the research that has been conducted using the core competency model as a framework for the research. Chapters 3 through 10 are devoted to each of the eight core competencies, with each chapter organized to present a synthesis of the research literature for that specific competency, research gaps that were evident in the literature during the years 2005 through 2017 covered by this review, and research questions that can be used to guide future research efforts on the role of the nurse educator. The final chapter, Chapter 11, provides insight into future directions for the nurse educator role and how the core competency model can continue to be used to influence future development of the role.

Over a decade after the core competencies were first published, the literature that is synthesized in this book continues to illustrate the complexity of our roles as nurse educators, the challenges that face us, and the rewards associated with teaching and influencing the next generation of nurses. This book is a valuable resource to nurse educators, novice and expert alike, as well as students engaged in graduate study who aspire to be nurse educators and are seeking a helpful guide to their own scholarship related to the educator role.

Judith A. Halstead, PhD, RN, ANEF, FAAN

Contents

1

The Influence of the Core Competencies for Nurse Educators: 2005–2015

Linda S. Christensen, EdD, JD, RN, CNE

Judith A. Halstead, PhD, RN, ANEF, FAAN

In 2007, *Creating an Evidence-Based Practice for Nurse Educators* (Halstead, 2007) disseminated the review of literature completed by the National League for Nursing's Task Group on Nurse Educator Competencies to support the development of the NLN Core Competencies for Nurse Educators and related competency task statements. The work of the task group started in 2002 and was completed in 2004. The task group conducted a comprehensive review and synthesis of the literature and identified the scope of practice for the academic nurse educator role. Its work was the foundation for formulating the NLN academic nurse educator core competencies and related task statements, the first evidence-based attempt to identify the competencies required of nurse educators to effectively fulfill their role. The development of the nurse educator core competencies has proven to be a seminal contribution to nursing education, serving to further guide the development of the academic nurse educator role in numerous ways.

More than a decade has passed since the original publication of the core competencies, but many of the forces that were affecting nurse educators in 2007 continue to impact the profession today. The continuing shortage of qualified nurse educators, along with the lack of a substantial pipeline of new educators to replace the large numbers of educators who are anticipating retirement, continues to be a serious concern for the profession. There also continues to be a shortage of doctoral programs that focus studies on the preparation of nurses for the faculty role.

In 2007, Halstead called for the profession to "focus attention on developing the next generation of nurse educators. It is essential that those who teach are well prepared to do so, and that they engage in an evidence-based practice of teaching" (p. 12). This call to action remains relevant a decade later. It is important that future nurse educators have the competencies required to effectively teach and practice in the complex and dynamic environments of health care and higher education. The core competencies and the updated review of literature that are presented in this book will continue to provide a framework of knowledge, skills, and attitudes that inform the educator role.

DEVELOPMENT OF THE CORE COMPETENCIES FOR NURSE EDUCATORS

When the members of the task group initially met to conduct a review of evidence-based literature and develop the core competencies and related task statements, they conducted their research based on a few guidelines and principles:

1. They were to address the question "What do educators need to know, or be able to do, to implement the role successfully and effectively?" (Halstead, 2007, p. 12).

2. The competencies were meant to address nurse educators who taught in varied academic environments (community colleges, liberal arts and comprehensive colleges, research-intensive environments, and clinical settings).

3. The range of experience and accompanying responsibilities of nurse educators across the continuum from novice to expert were to be captured by the competencies (Halstead, 2007).

The original task group conducted a review of published literature that covered the years 1992 to 2004. The intent was to focus on evidence-based literature, drawing from research literature in nursing, higher education, medicine, allied health, social work, psychology, and sociology databases. While the goal was to write an evidence-based synthesis of the literature, some of the identified competencies had little published research. Therefore, the task group had to incorporate publications that focused on best practices or exemplars into its work.

This current edition builds upon the foundation laid by the original task group. The authors of this edition began their review of the literature where the original work left off, covering the years 2005 to 2017, and using the same methodology.

The work of the original task group remains relevant both historically and contextually. The competencies continue to make a significant contribution to nursing education and the nursing profession, and serve as a guide to the continued evolution of the academic nurse educator role.

The academic nurse educator competencies were developed to describe the role of the nurse educator who practices in the full scope of the nurse educator role, incorporating all the identified competencies, including scholarship activities; service to the educational institution, profession, and community; and direct teaching with students. It is understood that there are academic nurse educators whose current positions do not require the performance of all the competencies. Indeed, when the competencies were originally developed, it was not anticipated that all academic nurse educators would practice in the full scope of the role, and that expectation has not changed.

IMPACT OF THE ACADEMIC NURSE EDUCATOR COMPETENCIES

It has been 13 years since the NLN published the academic nurse educator competencies (NLN, 2005). The competencies have been the basis for multiple activities since that time, including the development of nurse educator certification and research in the role of the academic nurse educator. They have also been used to guide role development and evaluation of nurse educators' practice in the workplace.

The NLN's Certified Nurse Educator® (CNE) program is the only certification available for academic nurse educators. Between 1999 and 2003, the NLN conducted two separate needs assessments related to the development of nurse educator certification (Ortelli, 2013). The decision to move ahead with the development of a certification program was made by the NLN Board of Governors in May 2003. The identification of the *Scope of Practice for Academic Nurse Educators* (NLN, 2005) supported certification development and became the basis for the certification examination test blueprint (Halstead, 2007).

The NLN Nurse Educator Certification program continues to operate as a semiautonomous department of the NLN with a mission "to recognize excellence in the advanced specialty role of the academic nurse educator" (NLN, 2012, p. 2). The NLN collaborated with Applied Measurement Professionals (AMP, now known as PSI) to conduct a practice analysis in 2005, based on the academic nurse educator competencies and task statements that were identified by the NLN's Task Group on Nurse Educator Competencies. This framework became the basis of a nationwide survey, which provided verification of the applicability of the competencies to the role through self-reporting of thousands of academic nurse educators. The practice analysis facilitated the development of the certification test plan blueprint.

The NLN piloted the certification exam in September 2005, with 174 academic nurse educators achieving the credential of CNE at that time. Since 2005, slightly over 6,000 academic nurse educators have demonstrated expertise in the role by achieving certification as academic nurse educators.

To ensure the test plan continues to be reflective of practice, the NLN, in collaboration with AMP/PSI, conducted repeat practice analyses in 2011 and 2017. These nationwide surveys of academic nurse educators continue to provide validation that the original competencies identified by the NLN task group continue to remain as relevant as when they were first identified in 2005.

Since the academic nurse educator competencies were first published, the NLN has received numerous copyright requests from nursing programs and faculty to incorporate the NLN academic nurse educator competencies within their nursing education programs. Many requests have come from graduate nursing education programs seeking permission to use the competencies as their program's curricular framework (program outcome competencies) for their graduate nursing education programs. Additionally, requests have been received to use the competencies within faculty position descriptions and faculty evaluation tools. Such use of the nurse educator competencies demonstrates how the evidence-based work of the early task group has been a positive force to shape and guide nursing education curricula and nursing education practice.

In 2007, it was thought that the identification of the core competencies of nurse educators would assist in the development of graduate nurse curricula and nurse educator practice, and promote the advanced specialty role of the academic nurse educator. In 2018, it can be said that the NLN nurse educator competencies have had a significant impact on the development of graduate nursing education curricula and nursing education practice. The competencies continue to address the challenges that face nursing education by providing "a framework by which we design a preferred future for nursing education" (Halstead, 2007, p. 14).

References

Halstead, J. (Ed.). (2007). *Nurse educator competencies: Creating an evidence-based practice for nurse educators*. New York, NY: National League for Nursing.

National League for Nursing. (2005). *The scope of practice for academic nurse educators*. New York, NY: Author.

National League for Nursing. (2012). *The scope of practice for academic nurse educators (2012 revisions)*. New York, NY: Author.

Ortelli, T. (2013). Evaluating the knowledge of those who teach: An analysis of candidates' performance on the Certified Nurse Educator (CNE) examination. Retrieved from Proquest (Dissertation No. 3617863).

2

Summary of Research Using the NLN Core Competencies of Nurse Educators as a Framework

Marilyn Frenn, PhD, RN, CNE, FTOS, ANEF, FAAN
Kristina Thomas Dreifuerst, PhD, RN, CNE, ANEF

Nursing education currently faces a number of challenges. The nurse faculty shortage continues to grow (US Department of Labor, Bureau of Labor Statistics, 2017) as experienced faculty enter their retirement years and the succession pipeline to replace them is limited in its ability to produce nurses who are qualified to assume the academic nurse educator role. As budgets tighten in higher education institutions, full-time tenured faculty are being replaced by higher percentages of nontenured and part-time faculty (Council for Higher Education Accreditation, Institute for Research and Study of Accreditation and Quality Assurance, 2014). These combined factors can lead to role strain among novice and experienced faculty alike and a continuing need to mentor and develop new faculty and larger numbers of part-time faculty. For nurse educators new to the academic environment, which differs from the clinical arena in which many had established expertise, it is important to help them understand their new role as teachers. Thus, the delineation of core competencies for academic nurse educators and the study of the effectiveness of approaches to improve nurse educator competence in the role are needed for the preparation and orientation of new faculty, as well as for ongoing faculty development.

The National League for Nursing Core Competencies of Nurse Educators©, first published in 2005, were based on an extensive review of the literature related to competencies of academic educators in higher education and two years of work by a task group of nurse educators (Halstead, 2007) to capture the competencies needed for success in the faculty role. The competencies (supported by 66 task statements) are:

- Facilitate Learning
- Facilitate Learner Development and Socialization
- Use Assessment and Evaluation Strategies
- Participate in Curriculum Design and Evaluation of Program Outcomes
- Function as a Change Agent and Leader

> ‣ Pursue Continuous Quality Improvement in the Nurse Educator Role
> ‣ Engage in Scholarship
> ‣ Function within the Educational Environment

Since their initial publication by the NLN in 2005, the core competencies have had a significant impact on the world of nursing education (see Chapter 1 for further discussion). In addition to guiding faculty development efforts and graduate curriculum development, these competencies also led to the development of the Certified Nurse Educator® (CNE) examination. The CNE examination was created to be a means by which nurse educators could be recognized for their "specialized knowledge, skills, abilities and excellence in practice" (NLN Academic Nurse Educator Certification Program, 2018). The CNE credential was also designed to be a credential that would recognize academic nurse educators as an advanced practice specialty (Ortelli, 2016).

Nurse educators prepare students for evidence-based practice, research, health care leadership, and the delivery of team-based, patient-centered care. Nurse educators prepare those who will be responsible for guiding the future evolution of the discipline of nursing. Examining the influence of the core competencies from a research-based perspective following a decade of use within the nursing profession is valuable to ensure that they continue to represent the complexities of the ever-changing health care environment while improving the preparation of the nursing education workforce.

Although little research was found regarding the use or testing of these core competencies in the review of literature from 2005 to 2017, it is important to note they were originally developed based on theory and best practices (Halstead, 2007) and continue to be validated through job analyses conducted with nurse educators (NLN Certification Commission, & Certification Test Development Committee, 2012). Moreover, the core competencies are an important framework by which to guide teaching practice and have been internationally cited as valuable by colleagues in Canada (Little & Milliken, 2007), as well as New Zealand, who have used them to examine the competencies needed by nurse educators in that country (Seccombe, 2009).

Despite their widespread adoption and influence since their initial publication, research conducted using the core competencies as a framework is not well known. Have these core competencies been used to guide nursing education research on the faculty role and responsibilities? What have we learned since the development of the core competencies? What research on the core competencies framework has been conducted, and what are priorities for future research?

REVIEW OF THE LITERATURE

This chapter examines the use of the NLN Core Competencies of Nurse Educators as a framework to guide research on the faculty role. The literature was searched using the Cumulative Index to Nursing and Allied Health Literature (CINAHL) from 2004 to the present using the following terms: NLN nurse educator competencies limited to English, Research, and also with subjects nurs** faculty competenc**, Faculty, nursing AND Competenc**. The search yielded 74 citations, but unfortunately, many citations related to nursing and student competencies; only one related to nurse educator competencies, and one related to health profession educator competencies.

The next search using National League for Nursing nurse educator competencies* yielded just four citations. It is significant that few studies related to the core competencies have been conducted since they were first published in 2005. As faculty continue to use the core competencies to inform and guide teaching practice, further studies specifically targeted to measure their use and impact are warranted, and peer-reviewed publications are necessary. Currently this represents a large gap in the nursing education research literature.

Searches using ProQuest Dissertations and Theses Global using NLN nurse educator competencies yielded 11 citations; the phrase "nurse educator competencies" yielded 114 citations. Education in ProQuest and Education Research Complete in EBSCO were searched using National League for Nursing nurse educator competencies* and one new study was found. The phrase "National League for Nursing core competencies for nurse educators" in each database yielded no new citations. All of these publications, as well as publications citing them, were carefully reviewed. Citations that were not empirically based or were not guided by the core competencies were excluded from the review.

Upon completion of the review of literature, there were three qualitative studies found that referenced the core competencies (Barta, 2010; Fox, 2017; Harper, 2017). Four quantitative studies were found that examined relationships with the CNE examination (Christensen, 2015; Lundeen, 2014; Ortelli, 2014, 2016). Six descriptive studies examined perceived competence (Higbie, 2010; Higgins, 2012; Kirchoff, 2010; Luoma, 2013; Poindexter, 2008; Ramsburg & Childress, 2012). Fitzgerald (2017) identified competencies included in graduate programs. And three quasi-experimental studies used a variety of investigator-developed instruments (Kalb & Skay, 2016; Mangum, 2013; Van Bever Wilson, 2010). Ortelli (2006) also reported the results of a national practice analysis for the CNE examination.

Qualitative Studies

Barta (2010) used a multiple case study approach to study the espoused and enacted teacher beliefs of four NLN certified nurse educators and the role they play in understanding relationships with nursing students. CNEs were challenged in their ability to engage students in the learning process, even though they felt effective in developing instructional pedagogy. Engaging students was challenging because human patients in the clinical setting influence the timing of teaching. Participants reported feeling different from colleagues at their educational institutions.

Fox (2017) used a naturalistic approach to examine the experiences of 14 nurse faculty new to a full-time academic role and their intent to stay in academia. Though the core competencies of nurse educators were referenced, only practice certification of respondents was reported. Fox found that clinical expertise was important, but not sufficient, for the academic nurse educator role and that participants were surprised by what they did not know.

Harper (2017) used a phenomenological approach to discover the knowledge, skills, and attitudes used in transitioning from novice to expert nurse educator. Having a structured orientation and mentor helped novice nurse educators. Being from a small school hindered faculty role development. Though the NLN core competencies were cited as a basis for the study, they were not addressed in the data.

Studies Focusing on the CNE Examination

The initial CNE examination, developed based on the NLN Core Competencies for Nurse Educators, was found to have internal consistency of .919, interclass correlation of .99, and at least initial content validity (Ortelli, 2006). As a measure of the core competencies from which research could be conducted, the CNE exam was developed and is regularly revised and updated based on job analyses; new items are continually developed by qualified, experienced certified nurse educators, and items are reviewed by nurse educators and experienced statisticians with measurement expertise, and the exam is administered under standardized testing conditions (NLN, 2017). The development of the examination, passed successfully by more than 6,200 nurse educators to date, is further detailed by Nick, Sharts-Hopko, and Leners (2013). Ortelli (2016) expanded this work by exploring the first-time pass rates of candidates on the CNE exam between 2005 and 2011; she reported an overall pass rate of 83.1 percent ($n = 2{,}673$), with the highest percentage of passing (93.9 percent) by candidates who had 21 to 25 years of full-time teaching experience prior to taking the exam.

Fitzgerald (2017), who reported that few published studies or dissertations were found related to the NLN core competencies of nurse educators, specifically focused on the CNE examination. She reviewed four studies (Byrne & Welch, 2016; Christensen, 2015; Lundeen, 2014; Ortelli, 2014) and examined the relationship between academic nurse educator preparation or experience and success on the CNE exam. Byrne and Welch (2016), who studied a sample of 20 full-time nursing faculty from one institution who had a preparation course based on the core competencies, found no correlation among the faculty role, differences in test scores, years of teaching, and the CNE exam pass rate. Ortelli (2014) reported a weak correlation between educational preparation and CNE subscores in three of the examination's test plan content areas: assessment and evaluation strategies ($r = 0.043$, $p = .03$); curriculum design and evaluation of program outcomes ($r = 0.040$, $p = .04$); and engaging in scholarship, service, and leadership ($r = 0.045$, $p = .02$). She also reported that those with an earned doctorate and those who taught in BSN or higher degree programs had the highest pass rates. Lundeen (2014) reported ($N = 390$) that most candidates who failed the CNE examination held a master's degree and taught in institutions offering graduate degrees, possibly indicating that they did not have experience with the full scope of the academic nurse educator role. However, Lundeen also found that performance on the exam overall, rather than certain areas, led to failure. Christensen (2015) found ($N = 795$) that total years worked as an academic nurse educator in an academic setting was associated with higher pass rates on the CNE examination. Given that competency is expected to grow with relevant experience (Benner, 2004), these findings lend validity to the CNE examination as a measure of the NLN core competency framework.

Researchers (Christensen, 2015; Lundeen, 2014) noted the lack of research examining the relationship of passing the CNE exam and student outcomes and faculty achievement in other aspects of the faculty role. Further research in this area may be possible as more faculty members achieve CNE certification. Similar to findings in nursing practice, where a 10 percent increase in BSN-prepared certified nurses was associated with a 2 percent decrease in both inpatient mortality and failure-to-rescue rates (Kendall-Gallagher, Aiken, Sloane, & Cimiotti, 2011), a critical mass of faculty who are certified may be needed to examine effects on student outcomes or faculty achievement. Studies that have examined the relationship of nursing education coursework to passing the CNE have the potentially unrecognized limitation identified by Fitzgerald (2017) that courses may not have included content relative to all the competencies included in the core competencies.

Higgins (2012) examined various evaluation instruments used to examine faculty competence, noting a lack of research with the NLN core competencies of nurse educators in the evaluation process of clinical nurse educators. The NLN has recently identified core competencies specific for the academic clinical nurse educator role (NLN Academic Nurse Educator Certification Program, 2018). These core competencies were developed using the same evidence-based methodology as the original academic nurse educator competencies and will provide the framework for an academic clinical nurse educator certification exam. *The 2018 Academic Clinical Nurse Educator Candidate Handbook* notes that is. Areas for further research include studies examining whether CNE certification improves faculty members' sense of empowerment and fosters retention, as has been found for certification in practice (Fitzpatrick, Campo, Graham, & Lavandero, 2010).

Descriptive Studies of Perceived Competence of Nurse Educators

Descriptive studies using surveys to examine perceptions of competency are another way the NLN core competencies of nurse educators have been studied. Poindexter (2008) developed her own instrument, based on the core competencies, to ask deans and directors (N = 374) to report minimal and preferred competencies of novice nurse educators. Cronbach's alpha was greater than .87 for all competency subscales. Competency was required for both tenure-track and non-tenure-track faculty members in facilitating student learning, facilitating learner development and socialization, using assessment and evaluation strategies, engaging in scholarship, and functioning within the educational environment. Competency was seen as needed for tenure-track faculty, whereas advanced beginner competencies were seen as needed for non-tenure-track faculty for participation in curriculum design and the evaluation of program outcomes.

Higbie (2010) also developed her own instrument to examine nurse educators' (N = 288) perceived attainment of the core competencies. Internal consistency was high, and correlations added to validity estimates. Power analysis indicated the sample size was sufficient to answer the research questions. Characteristics individually associated with higher mean scores were doctorally prepared faculty with greater than one semester of formal coursework in curriculum design, testing, measurement, and teaching strategies; being a CNE; and more years of full-time teaching.

Ramsburg and Childress (2012) asked 339 nurse educators about the perceived practical application of the core competencies using an investigator-developed instrument; results indicated that faculty characteristics with the highest self-rated levels of skill acquisition were doctoral degrees; working in a public university setting; more than 20 years of teaching and less than 10 years of clinical experience; more than 25 hours of professional development; and more than 19 hours of professional development focused on curriculum and instruction.

The relationship between formal preparation for the nurse educator role and perceived knowledge of the core competencies was reported by Kirchoff (2010) among newly hired (N = 69) nurse educators using an instrument similar to the one developed by Poindexter (2008). No significant differences in scores were found between novice (<1 year) and experienced (>1 year, average 5 years) nurse educators, or those with clinically focused master's and nursing-education-focused master's degrees. Areas in which faculty perceived themselves as less competent were engaging in scholarship, using assessment and evaluation strategies, and designing curriculum and evaluating program outcomes. No power analysis was conducted, and the study may have been underpowered to detect some differences.

The Clinical Teaching Evaluation (Fong & McCauley, 1993) was compared with an investigator-developed tool to measure perceptions of 35 associate degree clinical faculty members regarding meeting the NLN core competencies (Higgins, 2012). Clinical nurse educators evaluated themselves higher using NLN core competencies, compared to the evaluation given by their supervisor, in knowledge, t (34) = 4.4, p < .001, and competency, t (34) = 5.61, p < .001. Only three NLN core competencies were not used in the employer evaluation of clinical faculty members: (1) Participate in Curriculum Design and Evaluation of Program Outcomes, (2) Function as Change Agent and Leader, and (3) Function within the Educational Environment. No reliability data were reported for the investigator-developed instrument.

Luoma (2013) compared ratings of the competency task statements between 129 faculty and 14 administrators of nursing programs in one midwestern state based on novice-to-expert levels. The investigator-developed instrument used the task statements with Cronbach's alphas ranging from .91 to .98 for each competency. The same ranking was given for 22 of the task statements with no significant difference in level ratings for the competencies Facilitate Learning and Use Assessment and Evaluation Strategies. Two to four task statements were significantly different by one rating level for the competencies Facilitate Learner Development and Socialization, Participate in Curriculum Design and Evaluation of Program Outcomes, Function as a Change Agent and Leader, and Function within the Educational Environment. For the competencies Pursue Continuous Quality Improvement in the Nurse Educator Role and Engage in Scholarship, administrators rated half or more of the task statements more than two levels higher than faculty. Luoma recommended using the competencies for faculty development based on this initial study.

Quasi-Experimental Studies

Three quasi-experimental, pretest-posttest, no-control-group studies were found, each done at a single institution and each with a different investigator-developed instrument. Van Bever Wilson (2010) had 30 nurse faculty members rate their perceived knowledge using Kalb's Nurse Educator Self-Evaluation (NESE) an online survey tool based on the core competencies before and after attending a workshop designed to teach participants about the core competencies. The NESE, an investigator-developed instrument (Kalb, 2008), has been widely used. Cronbach's alpha was .798. With paired-samples t-tests, improved knowledge and improved ability to perform were found for 60 of the 66 task statements following the workshop. The design could be improved in subsequent studies, since this was conducted in only one school without a control group; nor was a Bonferroni correction used to evaluate the significance of the results for the multiple tests conducted.

The NESE, was also used by Kalb and Skay (2016) at the beginning and end of the nurse educator graduate program. Cronbach's alphas ranged from .75 to .94. Pretest ($n = 71$) and posttest ($n = 66$) data for students were not linked and only aggregate data were included. Significantly higher ($p \leq .001$) scores were found at the end of the program for student knowledge and skills ratings for all task statements, except Mentors and Supports Faculty Colleagues. Results should be viewed with some caution since data were from one school with no control group; moreover, an independent t-test was used, rather than a t-test for correlated samples, which is required when the same subjects are tested.

A three-hour core competency workshop was part of an evidence-based DNP capstone practice project with four newly hired faculty members. Faculty took a pretest and posttest for which Cronbach's alpha was .78 (Mangum, 2013). The Structured Orientation Development System (SODS) Nursing Faculty Self-Assessment Survey was developed by the investigator based on the NLN core competencies and Benner's (2004) model. One participant reported decreased competency following the workshop, while three participants increased their self-assessment survey scores. A paired-samples t-test did not show the differences to be significant, but the findings indicate that the SODS could be used as a structured orientation for new faculty members.

IDENTIFIED GAPS IN THE LITERATURE

Most instruments for which reliability and validity were examined had high internal consistency; the investigators found correlations with education and experience, contributing to the validity of the measures. Because instruments with acceptable estimates of reliability and validity are missing in many areas of nursing education science, further refinement of existing instruments is warranted. The use of self-report instruments regarding perceived competence is a limitation, especially since Gilbert-Palmer (2005) found that advanced practice nurses felt competent in five of the eight competencies, despite having no formal preparation for the academic nurse educator role or teaching experience. However, most of the APRNs studied were serving as preceptors, which provided them with some orientation and experience with these competencies. It should also be noted that Gilbert-Palmer's review was conducted in 2005, the first year of publication of the core competency framework, and dissemination and use of the core competencies were in the very early stages.

The results are inconclusive as to whether education, education with coursework related to the core competencies, or experience as a full-time faculty member contributes most to competence, though the weight of existing evidence favors years of full-time teaching. Those with doctoral preparation teaching in graduate programs did better on the CNE exam and rated their competence higher (Ortelli, 2016), but they were also the most experienced faculty members. A comparison of the findings since publication of the core competencies with prior findings was not conducted, though Gilbert-Palmer's (2005) review noted many of the same findings: educators with doctoral preparation perceived the competency of facilitating learning higher than educators with master's or bachelor's degrees. Those with more experience had greater teaching efficacy.

Others have used the core competencies of nurse educators, but not for research. For example, the core competencies have been used to develop curricula for master of nursing education programs (Kalb, 2008). Danna, Schaubhut, and Jones (2010) proposed a faculty orientation program based on the core competencies; it was based on their role transition experiences, not on research. Shelton and Hayne (2017) described the development of an online faculty evaluation tool using three parts, not the entirety, of the NLN core competencies: facilitating learning, facilitating learner development and socialization, and using assessment and evaluation strategies. Harper (2017) also noted that research on how to implement the competencies or whether they improved the ability of nurse educators was minimal. She aimed to study how the competencies were used to guide educators to acquire knowledge, skills, and attitudes in moving from novice to expert.

PRIORITIES FOR FUTURE RESEARCH

In summary, research using the NLN core competencies of nurse educators is in its early stages, and there are several priorities moving forward. First, there is little evidence that competency attainment impacts faculty performance and student outcomes. Research studies need to be designed that address this gap. Likewise, although some instruments have been developed that have acceptable estimates of reliability and validity, valid and reliable instrument development associated with the impact of the competencies is another critical research priority. Most of the few available studies have been descriptive and correlational, while the three small, quasi-experimental studies in this area have been single site, using a variety of investigator-developed instruments. As Schneider, Nicholas, and Kurrus (2013) noted, methodological rigor of nursing education research lags behind research in nursing practice. Therefore, not only would multisite studies with sufficient sample sizes, randomized controlled designs, and consistent instruments provide more substantive evidence, but also there would be opportunities for meta-analyses and rigorous conclusions—all critical for future research initiatives. Clearly, there is an opportunity going forward for much more rigorous research using the NLN core competencies of nurse educators.

QUESTIONS FOR FUTURE RESEARCH

➤ What valid and reliable instruments can be used in multisite studies (with sufficient statistical power to answer the research questions) to measure the impact of the NLN Core Competencies of Nurse Educators?

➤ Do the self-ratings of academic nurse educators' perceptions of self-efficacy with the NLN Core Competencies of Nurse Educators correlate significantly with interrater evaluated ratings of the core competencies?

➤ What are the priority competencies for nurse educators teaching full time in different program types—licensed practical nurse, associate degree nurse, bachelor's degree nurse, master's degree nurse, doctor of nursing practice, and PhD nursing programs?

> ‣ Which previously developed instruments with acceptable estimates of reliability and validity can be used in randomized controlled studies to examine the effectiveness of curricula developed using the framework of the NLN Core Competencies of Nurse Educators for academic nurse educator preparation?

> ‣ How can previously developed instruments with acceptable estimates of reliability and validity measuring performance of the NLN Core Competencies of Nurse Educators best be utilized in randomized controlled trials to examine the effectiveness of faculty development programs for academic nurse educators teaching in each type of program, such that meta-analyses eventually can be conducted?

References

Barta, B. L. R. (2010). *Certified nurse educators: Espoused and enacted teacher beliefs and the role they play in understanding relationship with nursing students* (Doctoral dissertation). Retrieved from ProQuest Dissertations and Theses database. (Accession No. 3438161)

Benner, P. (2004). Using the Dreyfus Model of Skill Acquisition to describe and interpret skill acquisition and clinical judgment in nursing practice and education. *Bulletin of Science Technology Society, 24*, 188–199.

Byrne, M., & Welch, S. (2016). CNE certification drive and exam results. *Nursing Education Perspectives, 37*(4), 221–223.

Christensen, L. S. (2015). *Factors related to success on the Certified Nurse Educator (CNE) examination* (Doctoral dissertation). Retrieved from ProQuest Dissertations and Theses database. (Accession No. 3708579)

Council for Higher Education Accreditation, Institute for Research and Study of Accreditation and Quality Assurance. (2014). *An examination of the changing faculty: Ensuring institutional quality and achieving desired student learning outcomes*. Retrieved from http://www.chea.org/userfiles/Conference%20Presentations/Examination_Changing_Faculty_2013.pdf

Danna, D. M., Schaubhut, R. M., & Jones, J. R. (2010). From practice to education: Perspectives from three nurse leaders. *Journal of Continuing Nursing Education, 41*(2), 83–87.

Fitzgerald, A. (2017). *Master's degree and post-master's certificate preparation for the academic nurse educator role: The use of the National League for Nursing Core Competencies of Nurse Educators as a curriculum guide* (Doctoral dissertation). Retrieved from ProQuest Dissertations and Theses Global database. (Accession No. 10260297)

Fitzpatrick, J. J., Campo, T. M., Graham, G., & Lavandero, R. (2010). Certification, empowerment, and intent to leave current position and the profession among critical care nurses. *American Journal of Critical Care, 19*, 218–226. doi:10.4037/ajcc2010442

Fong, C. M., & McCauley, G. T. (1993). Measuring the nursing, teaching, and interpersonal effectiveness of clinical instructors. *Journal of Nursing Education, 32*(7), 325–327.

Fox, A. S. (2017). *The experience of nurse faculty new to a full time academic role and intent to stay in academia* (Doctoral dissertation). Retrieved from ProQuest Dissertations and Theses Global database. (Accession No. 10277299)

Gilbert-Palmer, D. (2005). *Advance practice nurses' perceptions of Nurse Educator Core Competencies* (Doctoral dissertation). Retrieved from ProQuest Dissertations and Theses Global database. (Accession No. DP18426)

Halstead, J. A. (Ed.). (2007). *Nurse educator competencies: Creating an evidence-based practice for nurse educators*. New York, NY: National League for Nursing.

Harper, L. M. (2017). *A qualitative discovery of the knowledge, skills and attitudes used in transitioning from novice to expert nurse educator* (Doctoral dissertation). Retrieved from ProQuest Dissertations and Theses Global database. (Accession No. 10257661)

Higbie, J. K. (2010). *Perceived levels of nurse educators' attainment of NLN Core Competencies* (Doctoral dissertation). Retrieved from http://scholarworks.wmich.edu/dissertations

Higgins, T. T. S. (2012). *Evaluating competencies of clinical nurse educators in Associate Degree nursing programs* (Doctoral dissertation). Retrieved from ProQuest Dissertations and Theses Global database. (Accession No. 3522162)

Kalb, K. A. (2008). Core competencies of nurse educators: Inspiring excellence in nurse educator practice. *Nursing Education Perspectives, 29*(4), 217–219.

Kalb, K. A., & Skay, C. L. (2016). Revisiting the "Nurse Educator Self-Evaluation": Educating for excellence in nurse educator practice. *Nursing Education Perspectives, 37*, 307–309.

Kendall-Gallagher, D., Aiken, L. H., Sloane, D. M., & Cimiotti, J. P. (2011). Nurse specialty certification, inpatient mortality, and failure to rescue. *Journal of Nursing Scholarship, 43*(2), 188–194. doi:10.1111/j.1547-5069.2011.01391.x

Kirchoff, D. H. (2010). *The perceived role competencies and qualifications of newly hired novice and experienced nurse educators in prelicensure registered nurse programs: A regional study* (Doctoral dissertation). Retrieved from http://wvuscholar.wvu.edu/

Little, M. A., & Milliken, P. J. (2007). Practicing what we preach: Balancing teaching and clinical practice competencies. *International Journal of Nursing Education Scholarship, 4*(1), 1–14.

Lundeen, J. D. (2014). *Analysis of unsuccessful candidate performance on the certified nurse educator examination* (Doctoral dissertation). Retrieved from ProQuest Dissertations and Theses Global database. (Accession No. 3683685)

Luoma, K. L. (2013). *Nursing faculty professional development: A study using the National League for Nursing (NLN) Core Competencies for Nurse Educators for development of novice to expert nurse educators* (Doctoral dissertation). Retrieved from

ProQuest Dissertations and Theses Global database. (Accession No. 3597804)

Mangum, D. R. (2013). *A structured orientation development system for nursing faculty* (DNP Project Report). Retrieved from ProQuest Dissertations and Theses Global database. (Accession No 3589087)

National League for Nursing. (2005). *National League for Nursing Core Competencies for Nurse Educators*. New York, NY: Author.

National League for Nursing. (2017). *Certified Nurse Educator (CNE®) 2017 candidate handbook*. Retrieved from: http://www.nln.org/docs/default-source/professional-development-programs/certified-nurse-educator-(cne)-examination-candidate-handbook.pdf?sfvrsn=2

National League for Nursing. (2018). *Certified Nurse Educator (CNE®) 2018 candidate handbook*. Washington, D.C.: NLN.

National League for Nursing Academic Nurse Educator Certification Program. (2017). *Certified Nurse Educator (CNE) 2017 candidate handbook*. Retrieved from http://www.nln.org/professional-development-programs/Certification-for-Nurse-Educators/handbook

National League for Nursing Certification Commission, & Certification Test Development Committee. (2012). *The scope of practice for academic nurse educators* (Rev. ed.). New York, NY: National League for Nursing.

Nick, J. M., Sharts-Hopko, N. C., & Leners, D. W. (2013). From committee to commission: The history of the NLN's Certified Nurse Educator program. *Nursing Education Perspectives, 34*(5), 298–302.

Ortelli, T. A. (2006). Defining the professional responsibilities of academic nurse educators: The results of a national practice analysis. *Nursing Education Perspectives, 27*(5), 242–246.

Ortelli, T. A. (2014). *Evaluating the knowledge of those who teach: An analysis of candidates' performance on the Certified Nurse Educator (CNE) examination* (Doctoral dissertation). Retrieved from ProQuest Dissertations and Theses Global database. (Accession No. 3617863)

Ortelli, T. A. (2016). Candidates' first-time performance on the Certified Nurse Educator

Examination. *Nursing Education Perspectives*, *37*(4), 189–193. doi:10.1097/01.NEP.0000000000000024

Poindexter, K. A. (2008). *Essential novice nurse educator role competencies and qualifications to teach in a pre-licensure registered nurse education program* (Doctoral dissertation). Retrieved from ProQuest Dissertations and Thesis Global database. (Accession No. 3416072)

Ramsburg, L., & Childress, R. (2012). An initial investigation of the applicability of the Dreyfus skill acquisition model to the professional development of nurse educators. *Nursing Education Perspectives*, *33*(5), 312–316.

Schneider, B. P., Nicholas, J., & Kurrus, J. E. (2013). Comparison of methodologies quality and study/report characteristics between quantitative clinical nursing and nursing education research articles. *Nursing Education Perspectives*, *34*(5), 292–297.

Seccombe, J. (2009). What competencies do nurse educators need? *Nurse Educator*, *15*(10), 15.

Shelton, L. R., & Hayne, A. N. (2017). Developing an instrument for evidence-based peer review of faculty online teaching. *Nursing Education Perspectives*, *38*(3), 157–158. doi:10.1097/01.NEP.0000000000000130

US Department of Labor, Bureau of Labor Statistics. (2017). *Employment by industry, occupation, and percent distribution, 2016 and projected 2026: 25–1072 Nursing instructors and teachers, postsecondary*. Retrieved from https://www.bls.gov/emp/ep_table_108.htm

VanBever Wilson, R.R. (2010). Examining the effects of a National League for Nursing core competencies workshop as an intervention to improve nurse faculty practice. ProQuest Dissertations Publishing, 3409989.

3

Competency I: Facilitate Learning

Linda Caputi, EdD, RN, CNE, ANEF
Betsy Frank, PhD, RN, ANEF

Volumes can be written about how faculty facilitate learning, in part because of the complexity of nursing education. Nursing education covers various levels of nursing, from practical/vocational nursing education through advanced practice nursing. Nursing students arrive with myriad characteristics and prerequisite knowledge. Therefore, when studying how nurse faculty facilitate learning for nursing students, rather than a "one size fits all approach," faculty must consider a number of variables prior to determining an approach that best fits the level of nursing, content to be taught, level of thinking expected, and numerous student characteristics. The many task statements under the core competency Facilitate Learning reinforce this reality.

With all these variables to consider, there remains more that unites nurse educators across the academic continuum of nursing education than divides them. The literature reviewed demonstrates that no matter what type of nursing education the authors are addressing, their findings can be applied, although often with modification, to all of nursing education. This is important to keep in mind as nurse educators work together as colleagues across programs, schools, regions of the country, and internationally.

Competency I, Facilitate Learning, has a large number of competency statements. The following competency statements include the knowledge, skills, and attributes nurse educators must develop to facilitate learning effectively. The nurse educator

- implements a variety of teaching strategies appropriate to learner needs, desired learner outcomes, content, and context;
- grounds teaching strategies in educational theory and evidence-based teaching practices;
- recognizes multicultural, gender, and experiential influences on teaching and learning;
- engages in self-reflection and continued learning to improve teaching practices that facilitate learning;
- uses information technologies skillfully to support the teaching/learning process;
- practices skilled oral, written, and electronic communication that reflects an awareness of self and others, along with an ability to convey ideas in a variety of contexts;

> models critical and reflective thinking;

> creates opportunities for learners to develop their critical thinking and critical reasoning skills;

> shows enthusiasm for teaching, learning, and nursing that inspires and motivates students;

> demonstrates interest in and respect for learners;

> uses personal attributes (e.g., caring, confidence, patience, integrity, and flexibility) that facilitate learning;

> develops collegial working relationships with students, faculty colleagues, and clinical agency personnel to promote positive learning environments;

> maintains the professional practice knowledge base needed to help learners prepare for contemporary nursing practice; and

> serves as a role model of professional nursing.

For the purposes of this chapter, these competency statements are grouped into three categories based on common themes. This chapter is organized around those three common themes: (1) developing and using teaching/learning strategies, (2) creating an environment that facilitates learning, and (3) engaging in self-development to successfully and effectively facilitate learning.

REVIEW OF LITERATURE

The following databases were searched individually and together: Education Resources Information Center (ERIC), PsycARTICLES, Cumulative Index to Nursing and Allied Health Literature (CINAHL), Social Sciences Full Text, and Academic Search Complete, Medline, and Dissertation Abstracts. All searches were limited to the period 2005 to 2017 and to peer-reviewed, full-text articles in academic journals. With the competency statements as a guide, various search terms were used. Specific teaching strategies were searched, such as flipped classroom, dedicated educational units (DEUs), simulation, universal design, concept mapping, clinical reasoning, preceptors, and service learning. More general terms, such as faculty behaviors and attitudes, emotional intelligence, teaching effectiveness, colleague relationships, and communication, were searched as well.

As a result of the search, gaps were identified in the literature. For example, links between faculty attributes and teaching effectiveness were largely missing. Comparisons of full-time and part-time faculty on a variety of competencies were also absent in the literature. Themes that appeared with increasing frequency over the years included teaching with technology, interprofessional education, and a change in terminology from critical thinking to clinical reasoning. Of note, a great deal of research and other information has been compiled into systematic and integrative reviews.

This chapter reports on select topics that emerged from the literature search that provided evidence to (1) support what nurse faculty are doing, (2) provide new approaches for established teaching/learning strategies that facilitate learning, and (3) offer new ways of doing that were not part of nursing education in the past. The chapter ends with gaps in the literature and priorities for future research.

Developing and Using Teaching/Learning Strategies

As nurse faculty plan strategies to create environments that facilitate learning, it is always important to keep in mind that learning strategies are one piece of the bigger picture of nursing education. When developing and using learning strategies, faculty must carefully plan teaching methods that focus on specific competencies students are to achieve in the nursing course (Oermann, 2016). Teaching with purpose is the overarching goal and one must ask, *What is the why behind the what?* (Caputi, 2017). The specific competency to be learned must always be identified, then evaluated if the outcome was met. That evaluation is not just for the short term, but for the long-term effect of the learning. Oermann (2016) cautioned that we must keep in mind the question: "Will they retain that learning beyond the course, and will it make a difference in their later practice as a student and nurse?" (p. 218).

Specific teaching/learning strategies that emerged from the review of research and related literature include active learning, the flipped classroom, critical thinking/clinical reasoning, clinical education, simulation, service learning, and technology. After conducting an integrative literature review of evidence-based teaching strategies in nursing, Breytenbach, ten Ham-Baloyi, and Jordan (2017) concluded that although some strategies increased knowledge more than others, all teaching strategies increased knowledge level in some way. The authors recommended the use of multiple, innovative, evidence-based teaching strategies for the best results and recommended more research to compare the variety of teaching strategies, as well as the best way to use the many teaching strategies available. The authors also concluded that although some teaching strategies for nurse educators were described, there was a lack of integrative literature reviews summarizing the best teaching strategies to use.

Active Learning Strategies

Active learning refers to learners being active in the classroom. The focus is not on the teacher but on the student. This is also known as learner-centered teaching. The focus on learner-centered teaching aligns with the shift from behaviorism to constructivism in nursing education (Ellis, 2015; Harrington, Bosch, Schoofs, Beel-Bates, & Anderson, 2015; Plush & Kehrwald, 2014). Constructivist learning theory refers to what happens inside the person, how people integrate new knowledge into their existing knowledge frameworks as they create their own understanding about what is being learned. This process requires the learner to actively process what is being taught in the classroom while still in the classroom. Active learning based on constructivist learning theory is the basis for conceptual teaching, which supports the newly emerged version of the current concept-based curriculum movement (Giddens, Caputi, & Rodgers, 2019, in press).

Sand-Jecklin (2006) studied the impact of active learning on baccalaureate nursing students at one large university. Students exposed to active learning teaching methods reported an increased preference for these methods after a semester of instruction; however, students exposed to traditional instruction (lecture) had a higher preference for traditional methods. Shatto, L'Ecuyer, and Quinn (2017) surveyed baccalaureate nursing students at the beginning of the semester after the first class when 46 percent of students reported they were "greatly satisfied" with active learning in the classroom; this number increased to 85 percent by the end of the course. Dabney and Mitchell (2017) reported similar results. Based on these findings, faculty encountering student resistance to active learning strategies are encouraged to continue their efforts throughout the term.

Many authors provide strategies to foster a learner-centered classroom with increased learning through active processing (Aljezawi & Albashtawy, 2015; DuHamel et al., 2011; Ferszt, Dugas, McGrane, & Calderelli, 2017; Herrman, 2011; McCulley & Jones, 2014; Smallheer, 2016). Active learning classrooms are applicable to all content areas across educational levels. For example, Nadelson and Nadelson (2014) described active learning methods used to teach evidence-based practice, and Wonder and Otte (2015) used active learning strategies to teach nursing statistics. Based on a literary review of teaching strategies in graduate-level nursing education, Duhamel (2016) recommended that traditional teaching approaches should be replaced with a learner-centered classroom to promote better, more creative problem-solving opportunities. Tully (2010) compared the use of inquiry-based learning to traditional methods of classroom teaching with nurse midwife students. The study used a qualitative phenomenological research approach to analyze the students' satisfaction with inquiry-based learning, the impact on clinical learning, students' motivation, issues around group work, and the role of the facilitator. The overall finding was that students were more proactive in their learning with inquiry-based learning, which resulted in a positive impact on their clinical practice. No further information was provided about what the positive impact was or how it was measured.

A pilot quasi-experimental study using 11 medical students in the experimental group and 14 in the nonexperimental group showed that active learning strategies were useful in improving identification of key problems. But knowledge gains demonstrated via a multiple choice exam showed no difference between students who engaged in small-group team-based learning versus those who didn't engage in team-based learning (Jost, Brüstle, Giesler, Rijntjes, & Brich, 2017). Perhaps active learning strategies are more appropriate when teaching clinical reasoning, but traditional teaching methods may be more appropriate for basic knowledge acquisition. Larger studies are needed to verify what teaching/learning strategies are appropriate for different kinds of learning.

The Flipped Classroom

The flipped classroom is a new approach to teaching in nursing education. With this approach direct instruction moves outside the classroom space in the form of preclass activities. Class time is then spent engaging in active learning strategies that apply preclass activities to creative applications of the subject matter, problem solving, and higher level thinking processes (Hessler, 2017). Hawks (2014) summarized flipped activities in the nursing classroom as "discussing points of confusion, providing real-life examples relevant to course content, challenging students to think more deeply about complex processes, and monitoring peer-to-peer, team-based learning activities" (p. 265). Njie-Carr et al. (2016) asserted the activities used in the flipped classroom are important to prepare students for the future workforce.

Although the flipped classroom engages students in activities, there are concerns about the approach on the part of both students and faculty. In an integrative review of the literature, Njie-Carr et al. (2016) found that student-related concerns included the time needed for preclass assignments and Internet access; faculty-related concerns included the time needed for the development of the flipped classroom course, the different student learning styles, and technology support. Future course modifications by faculty are expected to take less time to create and implement once the initial course is developed (Peisachovich, Murtha, Phillips, & Messinger, 2016).

Drawing on a review of evidence supporting the use of the flipped classroom, Hawks (2014) offered tenets of the flipped classroom, some of which include the following: (1) draws on active learning, student engagement, and hybrid course design; (2) blends direct instruction with constructivist learning; (3) personalizes student learning; (4) promotes deep learning; (5) builds on what students already know; and (6) supports collaboration, teamwork, and peer-to-peer mentoring. The instructor's role is to connect concepts and fill in knowledge gaps. The flipped classroom expands on the active learning approach by engaging students in active processing of facts, knowledge, and information prior to class, then applying the preclass learning to active application and higher level thinking in the classroom. The nursing education literature provides evidence of positive results using the flipped classroom in both undergraduate and graduate education (Critz & Knight, 2013; Missildine, Fountain, Summers, & Gosselin, 2013; Peisachovich et al., 2016; Shatto et al., 2017).

The literature revealed a number of articles based the authors' experiences and application of anecdotal literature that provide guidance for nurse educators in implementing the flipped classroom (Critz & Knight, 2013; Cupita, 2016; Jakobsen & Knetemann, 2017; McDonald & Smith, 2013; Peisachovich et al., 2016; Schwartz, 2014). For the flipped classroom pedagogy to be effective, faculty must accept this pedagogy as worthy of the time and work invested. In addition, faculty must prepare students for the flipped classroom (Hawks, 2014). Students who are accustomed to the traditional classroom may resist this pedagogy until they understand the rationale for this approach. Faculty must also plan effective preclass activities that support in-class activities (Critz & Knight, 2013). There are no specific preclass activities; rather, activities are those that best prepare students for the classroom. Activities may include recorded video lectures, specific readings, various written activities such as completion of worksheets or open-book quizzes, Internet searches for current health-related information, and a variety of other activities that are only limited by the creativity of the faculty and the purpose of the instruction.

Researchers who conducted literature reviews about the flipped classroom recommended further research on implementation of the pedagogy. Both Njie-Carr et al. (2016) and Bernard (2015) conducted integrative reviews. Njie-Carr et al. noted the lack of robust research on this topic, with the studies reviewed focused on methodology and process rather than scientific design. Bernard also found lack of rigor in the research studies. These researchers reported that the implementation of the flipped classroom varied, with classroom strategies ranging from well-designed and prescriptive to poorly developed activities that were not well explicated. Recommendations from these and other authors included evaluation of the process of implementing the flipped classroom and ongoing evaluation and refinement of the approach (Betihav, Bridgman, Kornhaber, & Cross, 2015; Presti, 2016). Njie-Carr et al. (2016) agreed with Oermann (2016) that further research needs to be conducted on the long-term effects of the flipped classroom; that is, will students/graduates be better prepared to engage in clinical judgment and decision-making months after learning in the flipped classroom environment?

Critical Thinking/Clinical Reasoning

Research conducted over the last decade supports a crisis in competency in engaging in clinical reasoning among new graduates. A national study by Del Bueno (2005) analyzed 10 years of results for more than 30,000 experienced and inexperienced registered nurses who completed the Performance-Based Development System. It was found that only 34 percent of new graduates were prepared to think at entry-level requirements. Twelve years later Kavanagh, and Szweda (2017) used the same system to study more than 5,000 nurses in Ohio. These authors reported that the number of new graduates prepared to think at entry-level requirements had fallen to 23 percent. All graduates studied in this research had passed the NCLEX-RN. Level of RN education did not impact the level of entry-level thinking. Clinical reasoning is a requirement for improving patient outcomes. If clinical reasoning is substandard, this could contribute to medical errors being the third-leading cause of death in the United States (Levett-Jones et al., 2009; Makary & Daniel, 2016; Purling & King, 2012).

Based on their research, Benner, Sutphen, Leonard, and Day (2010) called for a radical transformation of nursing education and asserted that newly graduated nurses are not prepared for the complexity of current nursing practice. Indeed, it is imperative that nursing students, in all programs, from practical/vocational nursing through graduate-level education, learn clinical reasoning applied to their scope of practice. However, a systematic, formalized approach to teaching thinking (critical thinking, clinical judgment, or clinical reasoning) has not been established in nursing education. According to Emerson (2007), "Nurses make thousands of decisions every day, and their ability to make those decisions is significantly grounded in their education experiences" (p. 483).

The literature revealed two distinct categories of learning related to teaching thinking. The first category relates to teaching the actual process of thinking, that is, how the nurse actually thinks while considering specific individual and contextual factors that impact the thinking required to arrive at the correct response (Caputi, 2018; Raymond, Profetto-McGrath, Myrick, & Strean, 2017). The second category is the application of the thinking process to patient care and other nursing situations.

Addressing the first category of developing a process to teach thinking, Tanner (2006a) provided nursing education with a research-based approach to clinical judgment that describes the four steps of the thinking process—noticing, interpreting, responding, and reflecting. It is important to note that Tanner's model is not the same as the nursing process. Tanner's model addresses the nurse's thinking. For example, during the reflecting stage, the nurse reflects on the thinking that was used and questions whether the thinking was effective or flawed, and whether another approach to thinking should have been used.

Tanner's model has been applied in nursing education by some nurse educators, but there is currently a gap in practice. Cappelletti, Engel, and Prentice (2014) concluded that Tanner's model needs to be extended, to move from understanding of clinical judgment to action; that is, education strategies that apply clinical judgment to clinical decision-making are needed. This is the basis for the Lasatar Clinical Judgment Rubric, which is used to evaluate thinking during high-fidelity simulation (Lasatar, 2011). However, a systematic, detailed process for teaching the process of thinking is lacking.

In an attempt to articulate nursing educator competencies related to teaching clinical judgment, Caputi (2016, 2018) developed the Caputi model for teaching thinking. It uses Tanner's four-step clinical judgment model with specific thinking skills and strategies included for each step. For example, thinking skills, such as differentiating important from unimportant information and deciding how much ambiguity can be tolerated in a situation, are examples of thinking skills used in the interpreting step. Learning these specific thinking skills applied to nursing practice sets the foundation for all faculty to formulate higher level thinking questions throughout the nursing program. Applying Tanner's model, Caputi's thinking skills and strategies, and Benner's (2001) novice to expert theory, Caputi (2018) provides an approach for teaching thinking across a nursing program that addresses the need to teach students how to link context and thinking with nursing-specific knowledge. Further research is needed to determine how these applications and others are used to improve the education of students (Raymond et al., 2017).

The second category of teaching thinking in nursing addresses a major weakness with the application of thinking, once the thinking process used in nursing has been taught. The expectation that students can apply thinking without first learning the detailed process of thinking in nursing has been part of nursing education for decades, primarily through the use of case studies in the classroom, care plans in the clinical setting, and debriefing after a high-fidelity simulation experience. Strategies to engage students in the application of thinking are necessary as faculty guide students through clinical decision-making. Forneris et al. (2015) used a quasi-experimental, pretest-posttest, repeated measure research design to study the use of structured debriefing following simulation to enhance clinical reasoning scores. The Health Sciences Reasoning test was used to evaluate nursing students' clinical reasoning. The results indicated that students who had the structured debriefing scored significantly higher in their clinical reasoning than students exposed to customary debriefing. Gholami et al. (2016) compared the effects of problem-based learning with the lecture method on students' ability to use critical thinking skills. The researchers used a quasi-experimental, single-group, pretest-posttest design with third-year nursing students and found a significant increase in critical thinking scores in students who experienced problem-based learning. There were no significant changes for students in the lecture group. The researchers cautioned that the management of the class and the details of the teaching strategies used in problem-based learning are essential components of this methodology. The specific teaching strategies that work best require further research.

Concept or mind mapping continues to be studied in nursing education as a method for promoting critical thinking abilities. Concept mapping is used at both the undergraduate and graduate levels as a way to determine how students are thinking. Clayton (2006) reported that a review of the literature demonstrated that using concept mapping assists faculty in preparing graduates to think critically in complex health care environments. Conceicao and Taylor (2007) conducted qualitative research through an examination of self-reflection journals of 21 students in an online course. The journals revealed that using concept maps helped students expand their knowledge base consistent with constructivist learning theory.

There are many types of maps and ways maps are used to facilitate learning. To truly study the critical thinking the student is actually using, students construct their own maps to demonstrate the cognitive connections they are making. Faculty then review these maps with students to determine and correct faulty thinking (Caputi & Blach, 2008) and demonstrate how the student constructs knowledge (Conceicao & Taylor, 2007). Faculty use these maps in the classroom, in the clinical setting, online, or in any educational environment for the purpose of analyzing students' thinking. Samawi, Miller, and Haras (2014) studied the use of concept maps to examine students' ability to critically ana-lyze a scenario, then apply theory to care of a pediatric simulation patient. Forty-eight students completed a simulation, created concept maps, and participated in informal focus groups. Their results indicated that concept maps used in simulation facilitated a deeper understanding of pathophysiology.

Clinical Education

The need to change clinical education, especially in prelicensure programs, is well estab-lished in the nursing education literature (Ard & Valiga, 2009; Benner et al., 2010; Ironside & McNelis, 2012; McNelis et al., 2014; Tanner, 2008, 2010). Most clinical assignments are based on a clinical model that has been in place for 40 years (Tanner, 2006b). Tanner (2008) stated, "The traditional clinical education model is taxing faculty, facilities, students, and staff, and increasingly relies on the availability of clinical placements" (p. 3). The Institute of Medicine's (IOM) 2010 *Forum on the Future of Nursing Education* called for nursing to "invest in a national initia-tive to develop and evaluate new approaches to prelicensure clinical education, including a required postgraduate residency under a restricted license" (p. 33).

The traditional clinical education model widely used in today's nursing programs is demanding on many levels but not necessarily effective (Gubrud-Howe & Schoessler, 2008). The IOM (2011) *Future of Nursing* report revealed that many of the hours spent in clinical settings fail to result in productive learning among students. Although students spend much time in clinical, performing routine care tasks repeatedly, that does not contribute significantly to increased learning, and little time is focused on fostering clinical reason-ing skills. Benner et al. (2010) noted that nursing relies on situated cognition and action and there should be a direct application of what is learned in theory sessions to learning in the clinical setting. Research conducted by McNelis et al. (2014) confirmed the IOM's find-ings. These researchers studied the clinical activities of 30 baccalaureate students in three US universities and found that a major focus of faculty was on students getting the work done. The work most frequently done by nursing students was predominantly routine hygiene, vital signs, and medication administration, with missed opportunities to engage in more complex aspects of nursing practice.

Although requests for change have been issued for the last 15 years, only a few models have been offered to change the age-old clinical model for all levels of nursing education. These include the establishment of DEUs, a focus on critical thinking/clinical reasoning through changes in clinical day assignments, and the use of simulation as a substitute for clinical experience.

The IOM (2011) *Future of Nursing* report recommends the use of DEUs as a means for expanding clinical capacity. With DEUs, staff nurses serve as clinical educators and are provided mentoring and education in this role. Faculty serve as mentors and facilitate a community of learning on the unit (Bower, Swoboda, & Jeffries, 2014). This model represents a change in academic and practice partnerships (Dapremont & Lee, 2013). The unit staff and faculty work in a close partnership to facilitate clinical learning. Estab-lishing role responsibilities is important with the DEU model. DeMeester (2016) reported that faculty need to have a purpose in their teaching role with this model. Glynn, McVey, Wendt, and Russell (2017) researched DEUs and recommended that caseloads for staff nurses serving as clinical instructors be less when students are present, requiring a commitment from the practice institution. However, having time to teach was reported by staff nurses as an important factor when working with students, even in a non-DEU unit (Rebeiro, Edward, Chapman, & Evans, 2015). Rebeiro et al. conducted an integrative review of the literature relating to clinical instruction and reported other important issues that must be addressed, including (1) communication about how to merge theory with practice, (2) structured orientation to the role with clear clinical objectives, (3) information about meeting the learning needs for diverse learners and those needing accommodations, (4) recognition for their role as clinical instructor with feedback to promote growth in the role, and (5) how to promote the students' ability to engage in critical thinking. The researchers noted the need for further research in the area of developing critical thinking on the DEU.

Jeffries et al. (2013) researched a redesign of the DEU to develop a clinical academic-practice partnership (CAPP); the goal was to maximize the expertise of staff nurses and faculty and create a synergistic environment. The faculty role focused on working with students to integrate thinking and problem solving in the clinical practice environment throughout the clinical day while staff nurses were actively engaged with students. Preliminary findings of this study indicate that the students' sense of belonging is a key indicator of a positive clinical experience. Faculty and preceptors must create positive learning environments to enhance the value of clinical experiences.

DEUs have been the focus of a number of research studies over the last 10 years (DeMeester, 2016; George, Locasto, Pyo, & Cline, 2017; Glynn et al., 2017; Jeffries et al., 2013; Mulready-Shick & Flanagan, 2014; Nishioka, Coe, Hanita, & Moscato, 2014; Rhodes, Meyers, & Underhill, 2012; Sharpnack, Koppelman, & Fellows, 2014). George et al. (2017) measured preclinical and postclinical student self-efficacy, then compared students who had a traditional experience to students on a DEU. Self-efficacy, the belief in one's ability to plan and execute a course of action that will lead to the desired results, may be helpful in transitioning to the graduate nurse role. The self-efficacy of students on the DEU was significantly greater than that of the traditional students. Their ability to actually plan and execute a course of action was not measured.

DeMeester's (2016) research revealed that students frequently questioned the care they observed while working on a DEU. DeMeester recommended that faculty play a role in helping students think through practice issues and how to improve and support evidence-based practice. Sharpnack et al. (2014) researched the effectiveness of DEUs with second-degree accelerated nursing students. They reported that after graduation, the DEU students were hired by the units where they spent their clinical time, reducing the time allotted for orientation and improving retention, both positive outcomes for the practice partner. Research by Mulready-Shick and Flanagan (2014) revealed that sustainability of DEUs is dependent on nurturing the role of the staff nurses serving as preceptors. Critical to this process is the fostering of the relationship among all participants.

Caputi (2010) offered a new approach to teaching in the clinical area that addresses some of the IOM's (2011) concerns. One half of the group of students on a clinical unit is assigned to traditional patient care; repetitive, lower level nursing tasks are not included, and the focus is on the higher level thinking role of the nurse. While performing patient care and oversight of unlicensed assistive personnel, students also engage in deliberate recording of their thinking guided by specially designed activities. The other students in the group work in pairs and engage in critical thinking with a focus on patient inter-actions and specific clinical reasoning activities. Barrett, Krieg, Kinney, Maurer, and McKnight (2014) conducted research using the Caputi model. On a critical thinking exam, students learning with this clinical model outscored the previous class, which took the same criti-cal thinking exam, by 5 percent. The only change in the curriculum was the change in the approach to facilitating learning in the clinical setting. Faculty also reported a differ-ence in the quality of care and prioritization of care in the clinical setting and higher level dialogue during class activities.

Gazarian and Pennington (2012) implemented a unique approach to learning in the clinical setting. At the beginning of a classroom session an expert nurse from the clinical setting provides a shift report on the patients being cared for on that shift. During the classroom time faculty and students process this information; clarify terms and identify missing information; and reinforce textbook knowledge and how it relates to the reported clinical situation. The faculty member then guides the students to deeper learning by probing various clinical patient situations through strategies such as students posing questions directly related to the report and planning care. At the end of the class session the expert nurse makes a second telephone call to the class. Students ask questions and the nurse talks about how the clinical situation unfolded throughout the time the stu-dents were in class. In a focus group conducted one month after graduation students shared the relevance of this learning based on real patients by a real nurse in real time. Throughout the course nurses from various units participated in this classroom activity, providing the opportunity for students to discuss subtle differences among practice environments and patient contexts. The researchers described the classroom as chang-ing from a "place where knowledge is acquired to a place where knowledge is trans-lated from and applied to practice" (p. 215).

The common practice of students gathering patient information and completing paperwork the evening before clinical was the focus of two studies (Turner & Keeler, 2015; White, 2006). These researchers reported that preparation prior to the clinical day often resulted in lack of sleep and increased stress for students. In place of students preparing prior to clinical, students received individual assignments and reviewed the information prior to providing care on the clinical day. Students located and reviewed information as it was needed throughout the day. White reported students were able to complete all aspects of patient care and passed the clinical portion of the course. Staff and patient expectations were also met. Turner and Keeler reported no significant differences in clinical activities between those who completed preclinical assignments and those who did not; however, student stress was decreased.

The clinical postconference has been used for more than 40 years in nursing educa-tion. Megel, Nelson, Black, Vogel, and Uphoff (2013) studied survey results of the perceptions of the clinical postconference of 136 BSN students and 42 faculty. They reported no differences in student and faculty perceptions of the importance and use of the post-conference as a learning environment. However, the lowest scores from students were on the use of innovation, suggesting that postconference learning experiences might be enriched with increased use of active learning strategies. The lack of active learn-ing reported in this study might be enhanced with a focus on debriefing across the curriculum as outlined by the National League for Nursing (NLN, 2015), where the clinical post-conference is reframed as a debriefing session. Fey (2014) reported that only 31 percent of schools studied used a model to guide debriefing and less than half of all facilitators had any training. These results were based on a study of debriefing skills of simulation faculty; there have been no studies on the framework used by, or debriefing skills of, clinical faculty. The NLN recommended debriefing across the curriculum, including the clinical setting. The use of skilled debriefing is an area of future research with the potential to greatly improve clinical learning.

Simulation

Simulation focused on a variety of topics is a widely accepted methodology for facilitating learning in nursing education (Cant & Cooper, 2009). Examples of simulation include the use of task trainers, role playing, static manikins, and high-fidelity manikins. Fabro, Schaffer, and Scharton (2014) studied the use of high-fidelity simulation to teach end-of-life care. Qualitative data about student perceptions were studied through an analysis of student reflection papers; results indicated greater student confidence and better preparation in caring for patients receiving palliative nursing care. Murphy and Nimmagadda (2015) used simulation that brought together nursing and social work students to address interprofessional education. Students from both professions improved their scores on the Readiness for Interprofessional Learning Scale.

Bruce et al. (2009) looked at intraprofessional collaboration by coupling graduate and undergraduate nursing students to engage in a mock cardiac arrest using high-fidelity simulation. Students scored higher on postsimulation testing than presimulation testing, although the results for confidence were not statistically significant. However, students at both levels of education reported high satisfaction with the experience of participating as a member of the team during a cardiac arrest.

Other authors combined simulation with other teaching/learning strategies. Sinclair and Ferguson (2009) studied the integration of simulation into the nursing theory classroom. The results suggested that students' self-confidence increased. Students also indicated higher levels of satisfaction, effectiveness, and consistency with their learning style compared with lecture as the only method used. Carson and Harder (2016) also studied the combination of lecture and simulation and provided suggestions for using simulation in a large didactic classroom setting. Shanty and Gropelli (2014) combined high-fidelity simulation with role play in a didactic classroom to simulate managing multiple patients with a role-playing application of leadership concepts.

Samawi et al. (2014) studied the combination of concept mapping with clinical simulation scenarios. Students self-reported that their self-confidence and critical thinking were significantly improved. Research conducted by Strickland, Cheshire, and March (2017) used the Lasatar Clinical Judgment Rubric to compare students' self-assessment of clinical judgment skills and faculty's assessment of the students' ability. They found students rated themselves higher on their ability to engage in critical thinking after a simulation experience than the ratings of their faculty. They concluded it is crucial that nursing educators directly observe, evaluate, and provide feedback to students. An area for further research is the development of a systematic, universal method for evaluating gains in critical thinking/clinical reasoning with simulation.

As with all methodologies in nursing education, faculty development is needed to receive the most benefit from simulation (McNeill, Parker, Nadeau, Pelayo, & Cook, 2012; Parish, 2010). There are a few credible sources for faculty development in the use of simulation. The International Nursing Association for Clinical Simulation and Learning (INACSL) has grown into a mature organization that provides learning opportunities related to clinical simulation, as well as a vision that includes research, evaluation, and integration of teaching strategies. The NLN published the NLN Jeffries Simulation Theory, which provides faculty with a research-based model for simulation (Jeffries, 2015).

Service Learning

Service learning is a strategy that helps students develop critical thinking skills in a large array of community settings (Arnold, 2014). One goal of service learning is to foster community engagement. However, Arnold's (2014) systematic review of the literature demonstrated only a moderate relationship between service learning and civic engagement postgraduation.

The literature in nursing education contains numerous articles about service learning pedagogy, but many do not report the collection of data to validate the outcomes of service learning. For example, O'Neill (2016) reported on using service learning connected to health policy in a senior baccalaureate nursing course. Her description was very thorough, but no hard data were collected to validate the efficacy of this approach to service learning. Kohlbry and Daugherty (2015) used some journal data to support the positive impact of an international service learning experience. However, other authors have presented more substantial data regarding learning outcomes. Collecting sufficient data regarding the efficacy of service learning as a pedagogy worthy of incorporating into the nurse educator's toolbox is essential.

Reising et al. (2008) conducted research on second- and third-year students. One hundred and seventy-three second-year students in a community assessment course collected health promotion data and developed and implemented patient education.

Then in a research and statistic course during the third year, they analyzed their data. Data from a pretest/posttest design showed that participants in the educational programs (120 in the heart disease education program and 214 in the diabetes education program) showed significant gains in knowledge at the p.000 level. Student data showed they valued the ability to see health promotion in action and agreed that service learning helped them to achieve stated curricular outcomes.

Groh, Stallwood, and Daniels (2011) collected data over a six-year period on 306 senior nursing students. Students engaged in 10 hours of service learning during one semester. Data were collected using the Self-Evaluation Service Learning Tool, which measured perception of leadership skills and social justice interests. All items on the tool, with the exception of care for self and others, showed statistically significant positive changes as a result of the service learning.

Technology

The term *technology* encompasses many varieties of technology used to facilitate learning. The literature revealed a number of research studies that focused on various types of technology. Montenery et al. (2013) researched student preferences for a number of technologies and found that students positively rated the use of audience response systems (highest ratings), virtual learning, and simulation as contributing to their class participation, learning, attention, and satisfaction. The participants also strongly preferred computerized testing. In an earlier study Revell and McCurry (2010) reported similar results related to the use of an audience response system. Students and faculty both reported the response systems were effective in promoting engagement, fostering critical thinking, and improving learning outcomes with both small and large classes. Berry (2009) studied the use of an audience response system to promote whole-class engagement in a course taught over interactive television (ITV) to two sites simultaneously. The response system was used to receive input from, and provide immediate feedback to, students. Final course grades were significantly higher for students using the response system compared to those of a previous class who did not use the response system.

Faculty also use YouTube to engage students with the intent of enhancing learning and improving retention of content (Wright & Abell, 2011). Zamora, Sarpy, and Kittipha (2017) used YouTube to promote engagement in learning and to teach difficult pharmacological concepts. Students were assigned a specific drug then developed a YouTube video for that drug. All students watched all the videos developed by their classmates. Students reported positive feedback about the assignment. Research related to the achievement of learning outcomes using this type of technology is needed.

A 2014 study looked at the effect of texting on students' perceptions of learning in an online course. Swatzwelder (2014) found that students using texting as part of the course requirements indicated a positive perception of learning; faculty perceptions of learning were also positive. However, there was no statistical difference in scores on graded assignments between the group that used texting and the group that did not use texting. The researcher concluded that both students and faculty agreed that texting is an accepted method for interactivity in the online course.

Research on newer technologies is just emerging, and more research is needed to determine the best uses and the most effective ways to use technology to facilitate learning.

Over the last decade online learning has expanded exponentially. Research-supported standards are provided by Quality Matters™ (QM) and the Online Learning Consortium (OLC). Skiba (2017) noted the importance of using research-based evidence to support best practices when developing online courses. A recent study indicated that following the QM guidelines for a large online course resulted in positive ratings by students about the design of the course (Crews, Bordonada, & Wilkinson, 2017). Skiba recommended that online teachers review the quality standards related to online instruction at their institutions and take advantage of the standards offered by OLC and QM.

Two recent studies looked at caring in online teaching. Plante and Asselin (2014) conducted a study that extrapolated evidence to support a social presence and caring online. Without face-to-face interaction with students, caring may not be evident. Their results indicated that faculty messages should be respectful, positive, encouraging, timely, and frequent to emulate caring behaviors. Additional caring behaviors recommended included caring interactions, mutual respect, and finding meaning in relationships.

Mastel-Smith, Post, and Lake (2015) also studied how to communicate caring in online teaching. These researchers sought to develop guidelines for caring online by studying faculty perceptions and expressions of online caring presence. They revised Watson's Ten Caritas Processes to apply to online nursing education and developed recommendations for an online caring presence based on these processes.

Creating an Environment That Facilitates Learning

A second theme to emerge from the review of research and other literature was the importance of faculty having the skill to create an environment that facilitates learning. Two subthemes were identified: establishing the environment and implementing strategies for specific groups of students.

Establishing the Environment

Studies continue to demonstrate that professor-student rapport (defined as "a relationship of trust and liking" [J. H. Wilson, Ryan, & Pugh, 2010, pp. 247–248]) supports student success through positive, enjoyable interaction and connection. Professor-student rapport has a number of effects including increasing academic performance, attendance, class participation, and student motivation (Benson, Cohen, & Buskist, 2005; Buskist & Saville, 2004; J. H. Wilson et al., 2010). Therefore, professor-student rapport is foundational to creating an environment that facilitates learning.

The topic of student-teacher connection was addressed by Gillespie (2005) in an article discussing the value of a student-teacher connection to create a transformative space for students. In this space students are affirmed, gain personal insights, and grow their personal and professional capacities. Likewise, Bryan, Lindo, Anderson-Johnson, and Weaver (2015) reported that students perceived the faculty quality of *realness* as a significant predictor of a positive interpersonal relationship between faculty and students. Realness is described as unveiling the "real self to the student without a front, facade, or any form of pretense" (p. 143). Realness conveys compassion, warmth, and understanding. This is especially important for male nursing students. Bell-Scriber (2008) reported that women perceived nursing faculty as more caring, connecting, and supporting than men's perception of nursing faculty.

One of the first encounters between faculty and students in which faculty can establish a student-teacher connection is through the course syllabus. Students report a preference for a longer syllabus. Saville, Zinn, Brown, and Marchuk (2010) reported that students perceived a shorter syllabus as an indication that the faculty member does not care much about them or their learning and is underprepared for the course. Students reported they would be more motivated to learn and more likely to seek help from faculty using a longer syllabus (Harrington & Gabert-Quillen, 2015).

In addition to length, a learner-centered syllabus provides a way to establish a learner-centered classroom and atmosphere from the start of the course. Richmond, Slattery, Mitchell, and Morgan (2016) researched student perceptions of faculty who created a student-centered syllabus as opposed to a faculty-centered syllabus as demonstrated by various syllabus components. Example components included accessibility of the teacher (only during prescribed office hours versus multiple means of access), collaboration among students (students advised all work must be individually completed versus collaboration through group work in class, discussion boards, etc.), and syllabus tone (punitive tone versus positive, encouraging tone). Students were asked to rate a hypothetical teacher based on review of the course syllabus. They rated the hypothetical teacher of the student-centered syllabus as more creative, caring, happy, and enthusiastic; willing to foster their learning; creating a more positive professor-student rapport; and more receptive, reliable, and fair.

Implementing Strategies for Specific Groups of Students

The literature offers many ways to promote a positive learning environment that considers individual student characteristics. These include approaches that address culturally diverse students, underprepared students, and millennials. The professor-student rapport literature intersects with studies of diverse nursing students. The college student population has become increasingly diverse, with 36 percent of postsecondary students reporting to be African American, Hispanic, Asian/Pacific Islander, American Indian/Alaskan Native, or foreign born (Baumgartner, Bay, Lopez-Reyna, Snowden, & Maiorano, 2015). Fuller and Mott-Smith (2017) looked at the perceptions of diverse nursing students and faculty about issues that affect progression through a nursing program. Students reported the biggest hindrance to progression was a lack of relationship with faculty and classmates. Based on the increasing diversity of the student body, this is an important area of nursing education research. Interestingly, the Fuller and Mott-Smith (2017) study reported that faculty found the biggest hindrance to be language proficiency. Henderson, Barker, and Mak (2016) looked at the issue of intercultural communication challenges in academia. They noted there are gaps in the literature regarding resources available to address intercultural communication.

Other studies over the last 10 years reported a lack of cultural competence in nursing faculty (Marzilli, 2016; Sealey, Burnett, & Johnson, 2006; Ume-Nwagbo, 2012; A. Wilson, Sanner, & McAllister, 2010), with the observation that more culturally competent faculty will be able to provide a culturally sensitive learning experience. Dewald (2012) provided a list of teaching practices that can be used to promote cultural sensitizing in nursing education for the purpose of creating a positive learning environment for a diverse student population. Dewald noted the need for further research to determine if these strategies improve learning outcomes and recruitment and retention of culturally diverse students. Morton-Miller (2013) offered some general strategies for nurse educators to use to become more culturally competent in their teaching. These include the following: (1) assess the demographic profile of your current students, (2) reflect on your own cultural histories, (3) role model a cultural curiosity in the clinical setting and demonstrate incorporation of culture into nursing assessments and interventions, and (4) make cultural competency a priority and discuss "hot button" issues such as immigration and how to balance cultural sensitivity with the myriad other professional issues in a nursing program. Billings (2015) offered additional learning strategies for culturally and linguistically responsive teaching grouped into categories related to learning style differences among diverse students and students with linguistic differences.

Another variable that contributes to diversity of students in nursing programs relates to age. Students in nursing programs can range in age from 18 to over 60. Generational differences in the way people learn are important considerations when creating an environment that facilitates learning. Since the first edition of this book, a new generation has entered higher education, members of the generation known as millennials, born between 1982 and 2002. Members of the millennial generation are known as *digital natives* or the *Net generation* (Skiba, 2010). As with previous generations (baby boomers, Generation X), they were raised with societal influences that may affect the way they learn. For example, they are very connected. Millennials born in the earlier years of the generation were raised on computer games and personal computers; those born later, in the second half of the generation, were raised on mobile technologies such as smartphones and tablets. All millennials share the characteristic of being digital natives in contrast to most faculty, who are digital immigrants.

The literature provided some anecdotal insight into how to facilitate learning for millennial students. Because millennials are heavily connected to technology, the most obvious influence would be to use technology. However, caution must be used so that the use of technology is driven by purpose (Caputi, 2017). Skiba (2010) suggested faculty ask themselves, "How do I, as an educator, use technology to enhance thinking and understanding and promote learning?" (p. 251). Skiba (2010) provided two themes from Brown (2009) that summarized students' views on the use of technology inside and outside of the classroom: (1) "Too much or unfettered technology is bad and directly hinders learning" (p. 252) and (2) "The use of technology should not come at the expense of personal interaction both in and outside the classroom" (p. 252). Technology should not interfere with student-faculty or student-student interaction but rather enhance it, and should be integrated with student engagement. An example provided by Skiba (2010) is that capturing an entire lecture as a videocast is not a good use of technology. This video becomes a talking head and does not support student engagement. Learning strategies that move from learning content to mastering content are preferred—that is, mastering how that content is used. The biggest lesson from Skiba's review of the research in 2010 is that faculty are not using technology effectively to help students learn. The shift from technology first to learning first is critical for more effective learning.

In addition to being technologically savvy, McCurry and Martins (2010) reported other characteristics of millennial learners as being confident, team oriented, achieving, pressured, sheltered, and conventional with a strong sense of self-worth. These students enjoy structured learning with frequent, positive reinforcement. McCurry and Martins researched the use of an innovative assignment for teaching nursing research to millennial learners based on the learning preferences of this generation. Learning strategies included collaborative learning, presentations by clinical nurse researchers from diverse clinical and professional backgrounds, self-evaluation and peer evaluation, joint assignments with the corequisite clinical course, oral group presentations and posters, and research grand rounds. Traditional learning activities for this course included textbook reading assignments, didactic lecture with PowerPoint slides, unannounced quizzes, an orientation to online database searching by the librarian, and an assignment of writing a critique of a nursing research article. The researchers compared course evaluations using a Likert scale. The millennial students in the experimental group rated the innovative assignments as more effective than the traditional assignments in helping them meet the course objectives. Generational characteristics are important factors to consider when planning learning strategies.

Engaging in Self-Development to Successfully and Effectively Facilitate Learning

Three task statements listed in this category of facilitating learning reflect the educator's self-awareness to maintain the knowledge, skills, and attitudes required specifically to facilitate learning. Self-awareness is critical for ongoing improvement as a facilitator of learning. The task statements that align with self-development include:

> Engages in self-reflection and continued learning to improve teaching practices that facilitate learning

> Maintains the professional practice knowledge base needed to help learners prepare for contemporary nursing practice

> Serves as a role model of professional nursing

Research that addressed these task statements is scarce. The articles that were reviewed focused on the faculty's awareness or lack of awareness related to their role and how to apply their role responsibilities. However, a scarcity of research does not mean self-awareness is not important. All advanced practice nurses must consistently reflect and self-evaluate, then engage in learning to maintain or improve their practice. Nurse educators must address both their clinical practice areas and their practice as academicians to maintain currency (Lachance, 2014; Leonard, McCutcheon, & Rogers, 2016).

First, nurse educators must be aware of, and competent in, all role expectations. Understanding the full scope of practice is essential. Salminen, Minna, Sanna, Jouko, and Helena (2013) noted the importance of developing and using evaluation methods that reliably measure the level of nurse educators' competency in the clinical practice area. The authors also emphasized the necessity of communicating and collaborating with nurses in clinical practice to best prepare students for current practice and to decrease the theory-practice gap.

Unfortunately, actual expectations and evaluation of novice nurse educators in academia are lacking. Additionally, new nurse educators experience high levels of stress and role strain as they assume an academic position with which they are not familiar (Poindexter, 2013). Poindexter (2013) identified essential entry-level nurse educator competencies expected by nurse administrators to teach in a prelicensure RN program using NLN core competencies of nurse educators to determine nurse administrator expectations; 374 nurse administrators from 48 states were surveyed. The research revealed that 83 percent of administrators in nontenure facilities and 89 percent of administrations in tenure facilities expected entry-level nurse educators to perform at the competent or proficient level of functioning related to facilitating learning. Specific expectations included having a working knowledge of education theories, teaching strategies, and evidence-based teaching practice. Novice faculty are also expected to know how to teach to diverse learners and promote an environment in which students are valued, respected, and appreciated.

Although novice nurse educators are expected to be able to facilitate learning, they may need guidance and assistance to develop in this role (Brannagan & Oriol, 2014; Koffel & Reidt, 2015). To meet the expectations related to facilitating learning, nurse faculty engage in self-reflection to continuously improve their teaching practice, maintain a professional practice knowledge base, and serve as role models of professional nursing.

New nurse educators may be uncertain of the expectations in their new position (Pennbrant, 2016; Poindexter, 2013). Knowledge of and understanding one's role as a nurse educator takes time. Self-reflection with continued learning increases the nurse educator's ability and confidence to facilitate learning. A self-reflection that provides various items about the teaching role and expectations can help new nurse faculty engage in self-reflection. Dahlke, O'Connor, Hannesson, and Cheetham (2016) developed a survey tool to research clinical faculty and preceptors' perception of their role. Hou, Zhu, and Zheng (2010) researched and developed the Clinical Nursing Faculty Competence Inventory. These types of tools can be modified for specific use by mentors to focus self-reflection and identify learning needs. This is especially important because many clinical faculty have no preparation for clinical teaching. Suplee, Gardner, and Jerome-D'Emilia (2014) reported that of 74 nursing faculty surveyed, 31 percent reported no preparation for clinical teaching.

Peisachovich (2016) investigated the expansion of self-reflection to what is termed "reflection-beyond-action." This type of reflection is used to unlearn, to critically reflect on one's knowledge and beliefs and consider how these factors affect one's practice. This is a new phase of self-reflection. Peisachovich suggested Tanner's clinical judgment model be extended to include reflection-beyond-action. With this process professionals reflect on the "unproductive nature of old knowledge or frame of reference" (Delahaye & Becker, 2006, p. 8). The notion of unlearning to design and create a new approach to teaching nursing is an important area of future research.

The importance of faculty serving as role models for students has been with nursing education for decades and continues as an important aspect of teaching (Davis, 2013; Felstead, 2013). Felstead captured the essence of role modeling with the key point: "Adult nursing students should not be taught to play a role but learn how to embody the nurse's role and be professional in all they say and do" (p. 226). Benner et al. (2010) noted that terms such as *socialization* or *development of professional identity* have been used to express this transformation. However, a more accurate term might be formation that "denotes development of perceptual abilities, the ability to draw on knowledge and skilled know-how, and a way of being and acting in practice and in the world" (Benner et al., 2010, p. 166).

IDENTIFIED GAPS IN THE LITERATURE

Areas representing gaps in the literature and needing further research include a focus on the effectiveness of varied learning strategies to achieve learning outcomes. Most of the studies referenced in this chapter measured student/faculty satisfaction or perceptions of effectiveness. The purpose of using teaching strategies to facilitate learning is to ensure achievement of the identified course and program learning outcomes. Lacking in the research are studies that determine if increased learning occurred as measured by the achievement of learning outcomes at the end of the course and over the long term. As Oermann (2016) recommended, researchers should measure the effectiveness of the learning strategies to improve the students' or graduates' ability to engage in nursing practice over the long term.

Research is needed to identify best practices to guide the use of various teaching/ learning activities. For example, what are the best strategies for use in the flipped classroom? What framework or model should be used to conduct clinical postconferences? What is the best use of newer technologies to support learning in a variety of educational environments? What is the effectiveness of concept mapping on the graduate's performance on the licensure examination and in practice?

There are also gaps in research related to the abilities and competencies of nurse faculty to facilitate learning. For example, can improving faculty's cultural competency result in better facilitation of learning? What are the expected entry-level competencies for faculty new to teaching? What are the best ways to support clinical faculty as they are learning their roles?

As noted earlier in this chapter, research linking faculty attributes and teaching effectiveness was largely missing, along with research comparing the effectiveness of full-time and part-time faculty in facilitating learning as described in the various competency task statements. Such comparisons might be helpful in guiding the creation of faculty development programs designed to help faculty increase their effectiveness in facilitating learning.

Lacking in the literature are studies that look at best practices for teaching clinical judgment. The research demonstrated that new graduate RNs are not prepared to work at entry-level expectations (Benner et al., 2010; Kavanaugh & Szweda, 2017). This is critical because of the potential detriment to patient outcomes and produces an urgent need to research the best methods for teaching the thinking processes used by nurses.

Clinical education (McNelis et al., 2014) has reached a critical impasse. The call for changing clinical education in nursing has largely gone unheeded (Ironside & McNelis, 2012; Tanner, 2006b, 2008), which may be attributed to the lack of a replacement approach. The literature indicating patient outcomes are not improving and continue to be a challenge for all areas of health care (Makary & Daniel, 2016) supports the need for research on how to best educate students in the clinical setting as a priority. This chapter discussed some newer approaches to clinical education, but much more research is needed for the purpose of improving patient outcomes.

Additionally, there is a lack of research on the best way to measure the achievement of clinical learning outcomes. Clinical evaluation tools have not changed, just as the approach to teaching in clinical has not changed for decades. There is an urgent need for research on the objectivity and reliability of evaluation tools and rating scales used to grade students in the clinical setting (Oermann, Shellenbarger, & Gaberson, 2018).

The call for change in clinical education is focused mainly on undergraduate education. However, there remains a critical need for research on best practices for clinical education in graduate and advanced practice programs. Research on debriefing for both undergraduate and graduate clinical education is a priority. Because the overall goal of nursing education is to graduate nurses who provide safe, effective nursing care, all research that studies the application of learning to patient care is a priority.

As referenced throughout this chapter, measuring the effectiveness of teaching/ learning strategies to effect achievement of student learning outcomes continues to be a priority. The interventions used to facilitate learning are only useful if they achieve their intended effect, and that intended effect is based on measurements using student learning outcomes. Accreditation agencies at all levels of nursing education—the Accreditation Commission for Education in Nursing (ACEN), the Commission on Collegiate Nursing Education (CCNE), and the NLN Commission for Nursing Education Accreditation (CNEA)—as well as the regional accreditation bodies at the institutional level, expect faculty to demonstrate that students are meeting the learning outcomes they are to achieve throughout their program of study. As mentioned at the beginning of this chapter, teaching/learning strategies to facilitate learning are one piece of the nursing curriculum. Therefore, a priority for future research is to validate whether teaching/learning strategies fulfill their intended purpose—student achievement of learning outcomes.

PRIORITIES FOR FUTURE RESEARCH

The following priorities for future research related to the competency of facilitating learning are recommended:

> What teaching/learning strategies can be used to most effectively teach the thinking processes used by nurses required for entry-level practice?

> Are there new clinical teaching models for prelicensure nursing programs to better engage students in complex patient care?

> How can educators partner most effectively with practitioners to facilitate student learning in the clinical setting?

> What is the best use of student time in the clinical setting?

> How can faculty engage students in higher level thinking in the clinical setting?

> What are the best practices for clinical education in graduate and advanced practice programs?

> What are the most effective learning strategies to use with flipped learning in both undergraduate and graduate education?

> What types of debriefing are best suited for simulation and clinical education?

> How can faculty best validate if teaching/learning strategies are fulfilling their intended purpose—student achievement of learning outcomes?

> How can faculty best facilitate learning in graduate-level education?

> What are best practices for using emerging technologies in the nursing classroom?

> What are the best resources for addressing intercultural communication among faculty and students?

> What knowledge, skills, and attitudes are needed by faculty to facilitate learning in undergraduate and graduate nursing education, especially doctoral education?

References

Aljezawi, M., & Albashtawy, M. (2015). Quiz game teaching format versus didactic lectures. *British Journal of Nursing*, *24*(2), 86–92.

Ard, N., & Valiga, T. M. (2009). *Clinical nursing education: Current reflections*. New York, NY: National League for Nursing.

Arnold, B. (2014). *Long-term outcomes of service-learning on civic engagement and professional nursing practice* (Doctoral dissertation). Retrieved from ProQuest Dissertations and Theses A & I. (3728107)

Barrett, A. M., Krieg, C. B., Kinney, S. J., Maurer, E., & McKnight, P. (2014). The clinical portfolio: A success story in critical thinking. In L. Caputi (Ed.), *Innovations in nursing education: Building the future of nursing* (pp. 95–98). Washington, DC: National League for Nursing.

Baumgartner, D., Bay, M., Lopez-Reyna, N., Snowden, P. A., & Maiorano, M. J. (2015). Culturally responsive practice for teacher educators: Eight recommendations. *Multiple Voices for Ethnically Diverse Exception Learners*, *15*(1), 44–58.

Bell-Scriber, M. J. (2008). Warming the nursing education climate for traditional-age learners who are male. *Nursing Education Perspectives*, *29*(3), 143–149.

Benner, P. (2001). *From novice to expert: Excellence and power in clinical nursing practice* (Commemorative ed.). Upper Saddle River, NJ: Prentice Hall.

Benner, P., Sutphen, M., Leonard, V., & Day, L. (2010). *Educating nurses: A call for radical transformation*. San Francisco, CA: Jossey-Bass.

Benson, T. A., Cohen, A. L., & Buskist, W. (2005). Rapport: Its relation to student attitudes and behaviors toward teachers. *Teaching of Psychology*, *32*, 237–239.

Bernard, J. S. (2015). The flipped classroom: Fertile ground for nursing education research. *International Journal of Nursing Education Scholarship*, *12*(1), 99–109.

Berry, J. (2009). Technology support in nursing education: Clickers in the classroom. *Nursing Education Perspectives*, *30*(5), 295–298.

Betihav, V., Bridgman, H., Kornhaber, R., & Cross, M. (2015). The evidence for "flipped out": A systematic review of the flipped classroom in nursing education. *Nurse Education Today*, *38*, 15–21.

Billings, D. (2015). Culturally and linguistically responsive teaching: Part I. *Journal of Continuing Education in Nursing*, *46*(2), 62–64.

Bower, K. M., Swoboda, S. M., & Jeffries, P. R. (2014). The clinical faculty role for a dedicated education unit. In L. Caputi (Ed.), *Innovations in nursing education: Building the future of nursing* (pp. 53–60). Washington, DC: National League for Nursing.

Brannagan, K. B., & Oriol, M. (2014). A model for orientation and mentoring of online adjunct faculty in nursing. *Nursing Education Perspectives*, *34*(6), 128–130.

Breytenbach, C., ten Ham-Baloyi, W., & Jordan, P. J. (2017). An integrative literature review of evidence-based teaching strategies for nurse educators. *Nursing Education Perspective*, *38*(4), 193–197.

Brown, M. (2009). Learning & technology—"In that order." *Educause Review*, *44*(4), 62–63.

Bruce, S. A., Scherer, Y. K., Curran, C. C., Urschel, D. M., Erdley, S., & Ball, L. S. (2009). A collaborative exercise between graduate and undergraduate nursing students using a computer-assisted simulator in a mock cardiac arrest. *Nursing Education Perspectives*, *30*(1), 22–27.

Bryan, V. D., Lindo, J., Anderson-Johnson, P., & Weaver, S. (2015). Using Carl Rogers' person-centered model to explain interpersonal relationships at a school of nursing. *Journal of Professional Nursing*, *31*(2), 141–148.

Buskist, W., & Saville, B. K. (2004). Rapport building: Creating positive emotional contexts for enhancing teaching and learning. In B. Perlman, L. I. McCann, & S. H. McFadden (Eds.), *Lessons learned: Practical advice for the teaching of psychology* (Vol. 2, pp. 149–155). Washington, DC: American Psychological Society.

Cant, R. P., & Cooper, S. J. (2009). Simulation-based learning in nursing education: Systematic review. *Journal of Advanced Nursing, 66*(1), 3–15.

Cappelletti, A., Engel, J. K., & Prentice, D. (2014). Systematic review of clinical judgment and reasoning in nursing. *Journal of Nursing Education, 53*(8), 453–458.

Caputi, L. (2010). Transforming clinical education: The Caputi clinical activities portfolio. In L. Caputi (Ed.), *Teaching nursing: The art and science* (2nd ed., pp. 216–240). Glen Ellyn, IL: Dupage Press.

Caputi, L. (2016). The Caputi model for teaching thinking in nursing. In L. Caputi (Ed.), *Innovations in nursing education: Building the future of nursing* (Vol. 3, pp. 3–12). Washington, DC: National League for Nursing.

Caputi, L. (2017). The why behind the what: Teaching with a purpose. *Nurse Educator, 42*(4), 163.

Caputi, L. (2018). *Think like a nurse: A handbook*. Rolling Meadows, IL: Windy City Publishers.

Caputi, L., & Blach, B. (2008). *Teaching nursing using concept maps*. Glen Ellyn, IL: Dupage Press.

Carson, P. P., & Harder, N. (2016). Simulation use within the classroom: Recommendations from the literature. *Clinical Simulation in Nursing, 12*(10), 429–437.

Clayton, L. H. (2006). Concept mapping: An effective, active teaching-learning method. *Nursing Education Perspectives, 27*(4), 197–203.

Conceicao, S. C. O., & Taylor, L. D. (2007). Using a constructivist approach with online concept maps: Relationship between theory and nursing education. *Nursing Education Perspectives, 28*(5), 268–274.

Crews, T. B., Bordonada, T. M., & Wilkinson, K. (2017). Student feedback on quality matters standards for online course design. *Educause Review*. Retrieved from https://er.educause.edu/articles/2017/6/student-feedback-on-quality-matters-standards-for-online-course-design

Critz, C. M., & Knight, D. (2013). Using the flipped classroom in graduate nursing education. *Nurse Educator, 38*(5), 210–213.

Cupita, L. (2016). Just in time teaching: A strategy to encourage students' engagement. *HOW, 23*(2), 89–105.

Dabney, B. W., & Mitchell, R. (2017). Flipping an undergraduate gerontological nursing course: Student perceptions. *Nursing Education Perspective, 38*(6), 340–341.

Dahlke, S., O'Connor, M., Hannesson, T., & Cheetham, K. (2016). Understanding clinical nursing education: An exploratory study. *Nurse Education in Practice, 17*, 145–152.

Dapremont, J., & Lee, S. (2013). Partnering to educate: Dedicated education units. *Nurse Education in Practice, 13*, 335–337.

Davis, H, (2013). Modelling as a strategy for learning and teaching in nursing education. *Singapore Nursing Journal, 40*(3), 5–10.

Del Bueno, D. (2005). A crisis in critical thinking. *Nursing Education Perspectives, 26*(5), 278–282.

Delahaye, B., & Becker, K. (2006). Unlearning: A revised view of contemporary learning theories. In D. Orr, F. Nouwens, C. McPherson, R. E. Harreveld, & P. A. Danaher (Eds.), *Lifelong learning: Partners, pathways, and pedagogies*. Keynote and refereed papers from the 4th International Lifelong Learning Conference (pp. 26–31). Rockhampton: Central Queensland University Press. Retrieved from http://eprints.qut.edu.au/6532/1/6532.pdf

DeMeester, D. A. (2016). The lived experience of nursing faculty in a dedicated education unit. *Journal of Nursing Education, 55*(12), 669–674.

Dewald, R. J. (2012). Teaching strategies that promote a culturally sensitive nursing education. *Nursing Education Perspectives, 33*(6), 410–412.

Duhamel, K. V. (2016). Bringing us back to our creative senses: Fostering creativity in graduate-level nursing education: A literary review. *Nurse Education Today, 45*, 51–54.

DuHamel, M. B., Hirnle, C., Karvonen, C., Sayre, C., Wyant, S., Smith, N. C., ... Whitney, J. D. (2011). Enhancing medical-surgical nursing practice: Using practice tests and clinical examples to promote active learning and program evaluation.

Journal of Continuing Education in Nursing, 42(10), 457–462.

Ellis, D. M. (2015). The role of nurse educators' self-perception and beliefs in the use of learner-centered teaching in the classroom. *Nurse Education in Practice, 16*, 66–70.

Emerson, R. (2007). On becoming a nurse. *Journal of Nursing Education, 46*(11), 483.

Fabro, K., Schaffer, M., & Scharton, J. (2014). The development, implementation, and evaluation of an end-of-life simulation experience for baccalaureate nursing students. *Nursing Education Perspectives, 35*(1), 19–25.

Felstead, I. (2013). Role modeling and students' professional development. *British Journal of Nursing, 22*(4), 223–227.

Ferszt, G. G., Dugas, J., McGrane, C., & Calderelli, K. (2017). Creative strategies for teaching millennial nursing students. *Nurse Educator, 42*(6), 275–276.

Fey, M. K. (2014). *Debriefing practices in nursing education programs in the United States* (Doctoral dissertation). Retrieved from ProQuest. (3621880). Retrieved from http://0-search.proquest.com.aupac.lib.athabascau.ca/docview/1545890423?accountid = 8408

Forneris, S. G., Neal, D. O., Tiffany, J., Kuehn, M. B., Meyer, H. M., Blazovich, L. M., ... Smerillo, M. (2015). Enhancing clinical reasoning through simulation debriefing: A multisite study. *Nursing Education Perspectives, 38*(5), 304–310.

Fuller, B. L., & Mott-Smith, J. A. (2017). Issues influencing success: Comparing the perspectives of nurse educators and diverse nursing students. *Journal of Nursing Education, 56*(7), 389–396.

Gazarian, P. K., & Pennington, M. (2012). Clinical teleconferencing: Bringing the patient to the classroom. *Nursing Forum, 47*(4), 210–216.

George, L. E., Locasto, L. W., Pyo, K. A., & Cline, T. W. (2017). Effect of the dedicated education unit on nursing student self-efficacy: A quasi-experimental research study. *Nurse Education in Practice, 23*, 48–53.

Gholami, M., Koghadam, P. K., Mohammadi-poor, F., Tarahi, M. J., Sak, M., Toulabi, T.,

& Pour, A. H. M. (2016). Comparing the effects of problem-based learning and the traditional lecture method on critical thinking skills and metacognitive awareness in nursing students in a critical care nursing course. *Nurse Educator Today, 45*, 16–21.

Giddens, J. F., Caputi, L., & Rodgers, B. (2019, in press). *Mastering concept-based teaching: A guide for nurse educators* (2nd ed.). St. Louis, MO: Elsevier.

Gillespie, M. (2005). Student-teacher connection: A place of possibility. *Issues and Innovations in Nursing Education, 52*(2), 211–219.

Glynn, D. M., McVey, C., Wendt, J., & Russell, B. (2017). Dedicated educational nursing unit: Clinical instructors role perceptions and learning needs. *Journal of Professional Nursing, 33*(2), 108–112.

Groh, C. J., Stallwood, L. G., & Daniels, J. J. (2011). Service-learning in nursing education: Its impact on leadership and social justice. *Nursing Education Perspectives, 32*(6), 400–405.

Gubrud-Howe, P., & Schoessler, M. (2008). From random access opportunity to a clinical education curriculum. *Journal of Nursing Education, 47*(1), 3–4.

Harrington, C. M., & Gabert-Quillen, C. A. (2015). Syllabus length and use of images: An empirical investigation of student perceptions. *Scholarship of Teaching and Learning in Psychology, 1*, 235–243.

Harrington, S. A., Bosch, M. V., Schoofs, N., Beel-Bates, C., & Anderson, K. (2015). Quantitative outcomes for nursing students in a flipped classroom. *Nursing Education Perspectives, 36*(3), 179–181.

Hawks, S. J. (2014). The flipped classroom: Now or never? *AANA Journal, 82*(4), 264–269.

Henderson, S., Barker, M., & Mak, A. (2016). Strategies used by nurses, academics and students to overcome intercultural communication challenges. *Nurse Education in Practice, 16*, 71–78.

Herrman, J. (2011). Keeping their attention: Innovative strategies for nursing education. *Journal of Continuing Education in Nursing, 42*(10), 449–456.

Hessler, K. (2017). *Flipping the nursing classroom: Where active learning meets technology*. Burlington, MA: Jones & Bartlett.

Hou, X., Zhu, D., & Zheng, M. (2010). Clinical nursing faulty competence inventory—development and psychometric testing. *Journal of Advanced Nursing, 67*(5), 1109–1117.

Institute of Medicine. (2010). *A summary of the February 2010 forum on the future of nursing education*. Washington, DC: National Academies Press.

Institute of Medicine. (2011). *The future of nursing: Leading change, advancing health*. Washington, DC: National Academies Press.

Ironside, P., & McNelis, A. (2012). *Clinical education in prelicensure nursing programs*. New York, NY: National League for Nursing.

Jakobsen, K. V., & Knetemann, M. (2017). Putting structure to flipped classrooms using team-based learning. *International Journal of Teaching and Learning in Higher Education, 29*(1), 177–185.

Jeffries, P. (2015). *The NLN Jeffries Simulation Theory*. Philadelphia, PA: Wolters Kluwer/NLN.

Jeffries, P. R., Rose, L., Belcher, A. E., Dang, D., Hochuli, J. F., Fleischmann, D., … Walrath, J. M. (2013). A clinical academic practice partnership: A clinical education redesign. *Journal of Professional Nursing, 29*(3), 128–136.

Jost, M., Brüstle, P., Giesler, M., Rijntjes, M., & Brich, J. (2017). Effects of additional team-based learning on students' clinical reasoning skills: A pilot study. *BMC Research Notes, 10*(282), 1–7.

Kavanagh, J., & Szweda, C. (2017). A crisis in competency: The strategic and ethical imperative to assessing new graduate nurses' clinical reasoning. *Nursing Education Perspectives, 38*(2), 57–62.

Koffel, J., & Reidt, S. (2015). An interprofessional train-the-trainer evidence-based practice workshop: Design and evaluation. *Journal of Interprofessional Care, 29*(4), 367–369.

Kohlbry, P. & Daugherty, J. (2015). International service-learning: An opportunity to engage in cultural competence. *Journal of Professional Nursing, 31*(3), 242–246.

Lachance, C. (2014). Nursing journal clubs: A literature review on the effective teaching strategy for continuing education and evidence-based practice. *Journal of Continuing Education in Nursing, 45*(12), 559–565.

Lasatar, K. (2011). Clinical judgment: The last frontier for evaluation. *Nurse Education in Practice, 11*, 86–92.

Leonard, L., McCutcheon, K., & Rogers, K. M. A. (2016). In touch to teach: Do nurse educators need to maintain or possess recent clinical practice to facilitate student learning? *Nurse Educator in Practice, 16*, 148–151.

Levett-Jones, T., Hoffman, K., Dempsey, J., Jeong, S., Noble, D., Norton, C., … Hickey, N. (2009). The "five rights" of clinical reasoning: An educational model to enhance nursing students' ability to identify and manage clinically "at risk" patients. *Nurse Educator Today, 30*, 515–520.

Makary, M. A., & Daniel, M. (2016). Medical error—the third leading cause of death in the US. *British Medical Journal, 353*, i2139.

Marzilli, C. (2016). Assessment of cultural competence in Texas nursing faculty. *Nurse Education Today, 45*, 225–229.

Mastel-Smith, B., Post, J., & Lake, P. (2015). Online teaching: "Are you there, and do you care?" *Journal of Nursing Education, 54*(3), 145–151.

McCulley, C., & Jones, M. (2014). Fostering RN-to-BSN students' confidence in searching online for scholarly information on evidence-based practice. *Journal of Continuing Education in Nursing, 45*(1), 22–27.

McCurry, M. K., & Martins, D. C. (2010). Teaching undergraduate nursing research: A comparison of traditional and innovative approaches for success with millennial learners. *Journal of Nursing Education, 49*(5), 276–279.

McDonald, K., & Smith, C. (2013). The flipped classroom for professional development: Part I. Benefits and strategies. *Journal of Continuing Education in Nursing, 44*(10), 437–438.

McNeill, J., Parker, R. A., Nadeau, J., Pelayo, L. W., & Cook, J. (2012). Developing nurse educator competency in the pedagogy of simulation. *Journal of Nursing Education, 51*(12), 685–690.

McNelis, A. M., Ironside, P. M., Ebright, P. R., Dreifuerst, K. T., Zvonar, S. E., & Conner, S. C. (2014). Learning nursing practice: A multisite, multimethod investigation of clinical education. *Journal of Nursing Regulation, 4*(4), 30–35.

Megel, M. E., Nelson, A. E., Black, J., Vogel, J., & Uphoff, M. (2013). A comparison of student and faculty perceptions of clinical post-conference learning environment. *Nurse Education Today, 33*, 525–529.

Missildine, K., Fountain, R., Summers, L., & Gosselin, K. (2013). Flipped the classroom to improve student performance and satisfaction. *Journal of Nursing Education, 52*(10), 597–599.

Montenery, S. M., Walker, M., Sorensen, E., Thompson, R., Kirklin, D., White, R., & Ross, C. (2013). Millennial generation student nurses' perceptions of the impact of multiple technologies on learning. *Nursing Education Perspectives, 34*(6), 405–409.

Morton-Miller, A. R. (2013). Cultural competence in nursing education: Practicing what we preach. *Teaching and Learning in Nursing, 8*, 91–95.

Mulready-Shick, J., & Flanagan, K. (2014). Building the evidence for dedicated education unit sustainability and partnership success. *Nursing Education Perspectives, 35*(5), 287–293.

Murphy, J. I., & Nimmagadda, J. (2015). Partnering to provide simulated learning to address interprofessional education collaborative core competencies. *Journal of Interprofessional Care, 29*(3), 258–259.

Nadelson, S., & Nadelson, L. S. (2014). Evidence-based practice article reviews using CASP tools: A method for teaching EBP. *Worldviews on Evidence-Based Nursing, 11*(5), 344–346.

National League for Nursing. (2015). *Debriefing across the curriculum* [NLN Vision Series]. Washington, DC: Author.

Nishioka, V. M., Coe, M. T., Hanita, M., & Moscato, S. R. (2014). Dedicated education unit: Nurse perspectives on their clinical teaching role. *Nursing Education Perspectives, 35*(5), 294–300.

Njie-Carr, V. P. S., Ludeman, E., Lee, M. C., Dordunoo, D., Trocky, N. M., & Jenkins, L. S. (2016). An integrative review of flipped classroom teaching: Models in nursing education. *Journal of Professional Nursing, 33*(2), 133–144.

Oermann, M. (2016). Thinking about teaching in nursing. *Nurse Educator, 41*(5), 217–218.

Oermann, M., Shellenbarger, T., & Gaberson, K. (2018). *Clinical teaching strategies in nursing* (5th ed.). New York, NY: Springer.

O'Neill, M. (2016). Policy-focused service-learning as a capstone: Teaching essentials of baccalaureate nursing education. *Journal of Nursing Education, 55*(10), 583–586.

Parish, B. (2010). Characteristics of effective simulated clinical experience instructors: Interviews with undergraduate nursing students. *Journal of Nursing Education, 49*(10), 569–572.

Peisachovich, E. (2016). Reflection-beyond-action: A modified version of the reflecting phase of Tanner's clinical judgment model. *International Journal of Nursing and Health Science, 3*(2), 8–14.

Peisachovich, E., Murtha, S., Phillips, A., & Messinger, G. (2016). Flipped the classroom: A pedagogical approach to applying clinical judgment by engaging, interacting, and collaborating with nursing students. *International Journal of Higher Education, 5*(4), 114–121.

Pennbrant, S. (2016). Determination of the concepts "profession" and "role" in relation to "nurse educator." *Journal of Professional Nursing, 32*(6), 430–438.

Plante, K., & Asselin, M. E. (2014). Best practices for creating social presence and caring behaviors online. *Nursing Education Perspectives, 35*(4), 219–223.

Plush, S., & Kehrwald, B. A. (2014). Supporting new academics' use of student centred strategies in traditional university teaching. *Journal of University Teaching & Learning Practice, 11*(1), 1–11.

Poindexter, K. (2013). Novice nurse educator entry-level competency to teach: A national study. *Journal of Nursing Education, 52*(10), 569-565.

Presti, C. (2016). The flipped learning approach in nursing education: A literature review. *Journal of Nursing Education, 55*(5), 252–257.

Purling, A., & King, L. (2012). A literature review: Graduate nurses' preparedness for recognising and responding to the deteriorating patient. *Journal of Clinical Nursing, 21,* 3451–3465.

Raymond, C., Profetto-McGrath, J., Myrick, F., & Strean, W. B. (2017). An integrative review of the concealed connection: Nurse educators' critical thinking. *Journal of Nursing Education, 56*(11), 648–654.

Rebeiro, G., Edward, K., Chapman, R., & Evans, A. (2015). Interpersonal relationships between registered nurses and student nurses in the clinical setting: A systematic integrative review. *Nurse Education Today, 35,* 1206–1211.

Reising, D. L., Shea, R. A., Allen, P. N., Laux, M. M., Hensel, D., & Watts, P. A. (2008). Using service-learning to develop health promotion and research skills in nursing students. *International Journal of Nursing Education Scholarship, 5*(1), 1–15.

Revell, S. M. H., & McCurry, K. M. (2010). Engaging millennial learners: Effectiveness of personal response system technology with nursing students in small and large classrooms. *Journal of Nursing Education, 49*(5), 272–275.

Rhodes, M. L., Meyers, C. C., & Underhill, M. L. (2012). Evaluation outcomes of a dedicated education unit in a baccalaureate nursing program. *Journal of Professional Nursing, 28*(4), 223–230.

Richmond, A. S., Slattery, J. M., Mitchell, N., & Morgan, R. K. (2016). Can a learner-centered syllabus change students' perceptions of student-professor rapport and master teacher behaviors? *Scholarship of Teaching and Learning in Psychology, 2*(3), 159–168.

Salminen, L., Minna, S., Sanna, K., Jouko, K., & Helena, L. (2013). The competence and the cooperation of nurse educators. *Nurse Education Today, 33,* 1376–1381.

Samawi, Z., Miller, T., & Haras, M. S. (2014). Using high-fidelity simulation and concept mapping to cultivate self-confidence in nursing students. *Nursing Education Perspectives, 35*(6), 408–409.

Sand-Jecklin, K. (2006). The impact of active/cooperative instruction on beginning nursing student learning strategy preference. *Nurse Educator Today, 27,* 474–480.

Saville, B. K., Zinn, T. E., Brown, A. R., & Marchuk, K. A. (2010). Syllabus detail and students' perceptions of teacher effectiveness. *Teaching of Psychology, 37,* 186–189.

Schwartz, T. A. (2014). Flipping the statistics classroom in nursing education. *Journal of Nursing Education, 53*(4), 199–206.

Sealey, L. J., Burnett, M., & Johnson, G. (2006). Cultural competence of baccalaureate nursing faculty: Are we up to the task? *Journal of Cultural Diversity, 13*(3), 131–139.

Shanty, J. A., & Gropelli, T. (2014). Using active engagement to teach leadership. *Journal of Continuing Education in Nursing, 45*(12), 533–534.

Sharpnack, P. A., Koppelman, C., & Fellows, B. (2014). Using a dedicated education unit clinical education model with second-degree accelerated nursing program students. *Journal of Nursing Education, 53*(12), 685–691.

Shatto, B., L'Ecuyer, K., & Quinn, J. (2017). Retention of content utilizing a flipped classroom approach. *Nursing Education Perspectives, 38*(4), 206–208.

Sinclair, B., & Ferguson, K. (2009). Integrating simulated teaching/learning strategies in undergraduate nursing education. *International Journal of Nursing Education Scholarship, 6*(1), 1–11.

Skiba, D. J. (2010). Digital wisdom: A necessary faculty competency? [Emerging Technologies Center]. *Nursing Education Perspective, 31*(4), 251–253.

Skiba, D. J. (2017). Quality standards for online learning [Emerging Technologies Center]. *Nursing Education Perspectives, 38*(6), 364–365.

Smallheer, B. (2016). Reverse case study: A new perspective on an existing teaching strategy. *Nurse Educator, 41*(1), 7–8.

Strickland, H. P., Cheshire, M. H., & March, A. L. (2017). Clinical judgment during simulation: A comparison of student and faculty scores. *Nursing Education Perspectives, 38*(2), 85–86.

Suplee, P., Gardner, M., & Jerome-D'Emilia, B. (2014). Nursing faculty preparedness for clinical teaching. *Journal of Nursing Education*, *53*(3), 538–541.

Swatzwelder, K. (2014). Examining the effect of texting on students' perceptions of learning. *Nursing Education Perspectives*, *35*(6), 405–406.

Tanner, C. A. (2006a). Thinking like a nurse: A research-based model of clinical judgment in nursing. *Journal of Nursing Education*, *46*(6), 204–211.

Tanner, C. A. (2006b). The next transformation: Clinical education. *Journal of Nursing Education*, *45*(4), 99–100.

Tanner, C. A. (2008). From random access opportunity to a clinical education curriculum. *Journal of Nursing Education*, *47*(1), 3–4.

Tanner, C. A. (2010). From mother duck to mother lode: Clinical education for deep learning. *Journal of Nursing Education*, *49*(1), 3–4.

Tully, S. L. (2010). Student midwives' satisfaction with enquiry-based learning. *British Journal of Midwifery*, *18*(4), 254–258.

Turner, L., & Keeler, C. (2015). Should we prelab? A student-centered look at the time-honored tradition of prelab in clinical nursing education. *Nurse Educator*, *40*(2), 91–95.

Ume-Nwagbo, P. (2012). Implications of nursing faculties' cultural competence. *Journal of Nursing Education*, *15*(5), 262–268.

White, L. L. (2006). Preparing for clinical just-in-time. *Nurse Educator*, *31*(2), 57–60.

Wilson, A., Sanner, S., & McAllister, L. E. (2010). A longitudinal study of cultural competence among health science faculty. *Journal of Cultural Diversity*, *17*(2), 68–72.

Wilson, J. H., Ryan, R. G., & Pugh, J. L. (2010). Professor-student rapport scale predicts student outcomes. *Teaching of Psychology*, *37*, 246–251.

Wonder, A. H., & Otte, J. L. (2015). Active learning strategies to teach undergraduate nursing statistics: Connecting class and clinical to prepare students for evidence-based practice. *Worldviews on Evidence-Based Nursing*, *12*(2), 126–127.

Wright, D. G., & Abell, C. H. (2011). Using YouTube to bridge the gap between baby boomers and millennials. *Journal of Nursing Education*, *50*(5), 299–300.

Zamora, Z., Sarpy, N., & Kittipha, P. (2017). Using YouTube in teaching pharmacology to nursing students. *Nursing Education Perspectives*, *38*(4), 218–219.

4

Competency II: Facilitate Learner Development and Socialization

Susan Luparell, PhD, RN, CNE, ANEF

It is broadly understood that nurse educators are charged with moving learners along a continuum, from a less developed novice nurse to one who is more developed, yet still a novice, ready to enter the health care work environment and practice safely within it. Therefore, the primary emphasis of learner development within nursing education traditionally focuses on how students learn to think and act like nurses. This chapter addresses many key considerations related to learner development in nursing, including the theoretical underpinnings of student development, academic advisement, working with diverse students, facilitating learning and the development of critical thinking skills, and professional identity formation and values acquisition.

Nurse educators recognize their responsibility for helping students develop as nurses and integrate the values and behaviors expected of those who fulfill that role. To facilitate learner development and socialization effectively, the nurse educator

> identifies the individual learning styles and unique learning needs of international, adult, multicultural, educationally disadvantaged, physically challenged, at-risk, and second-degree learners;

> provides resources to diverse learners that help meet their individual learning needs;

> engages in effective advisement and counseling strategies that help learners meet their professional goals;

> creates learning environments that are focused on socialization to the role of the nurse and facilitates learners' self-reflection and personal goal setting;

> fosters the cognitive, psychomotor, and affective development of learners;

> recognizes the influence of teaching styles and interpersonal interactions on learner behaviors and outcomes;

> assists learners to develop the ability to engage in thoughtful and constructive self- and peer evaluation; and

> models professional behaviors for learners including, but not limited to, involvement in professional organizations, engagement in lifelong learning activities, dissemination of information through publications and presentations, and advocacy.

REVIEW OF LITERATURE

To identify the contemporary evidence-based literature for the period 2005 through 2017, the following databases were searched: Academic Search Premier, Cumulative Index to Nursing and Allied Health Literature (CINAHL) Complete, ProQuest Dissertations and Theses Global, Education Resources Information Center (ERIC), Google Scholar, and PsychINFO. Search terms included various forms and combinations of the following: learner development, student development, nursing students, higher education, critical thinking, professional comportment, professional socialization, professional identity, learning styles, academic advising, civility, and incivility.

To capture and describe the most robust forms of evidence available, emphasis of the literature review was placed hierarchically on systematic reviews of randomized controlled trials, reports of individual experimental and quasi-experimental studies, and, lastly, descriptive studies. In some topical areas little or no research was identified, while research was abundant in other areas; inclusion of all studies was not possible due to space limitations. In these cases, attempts were made to best represent the breadth of the literature, the most recent literature, and the most rigorous study designs. As with the previous text, a large body of the literature in this area depicts anecdotal experiences or single-site, nonrandomized pilot studies.

Theoretical Underpinnings of Learner Development

According to Broido and Schreiber (2016), "student learning and development are neither discrete nor isolated events. Learning and development are ... complex processes across the holistic spectrum of cognitive-epistemological, intra- and interpersonal aspects of students' identities and lives, constructed and reconstructed in alignment with the world in which they live" (pp. 71–72). The desired outcomes of any nursing program exist within the more global purpose of higher education, part of which is to challenge students to "grow and develop holistically, with increased complexity" (Patton, Renn, Guido, & Quaye, 2016, p. 6) and to "adopt increasingly complex ways of being, knowing, and doing" (Owen, 2012, p. 17). Therefore, when considering learner development, nurse educators should consider this broader purpose and be versed on the theoretical underpinnings guiding student development overall.

From the social justice perspective, students have a right to education that respects and values their unique identities and experiences, that is effective, and that is culturally, nationally, and globally relevant (Broido & Schreiber, 2016), with the goal of such education being to produce global citizens who challenge barriers and create just opportunities for all. Toward this end, multiple theories of student development exist to guide higher education institutions and faculty in both large- and small-scale efforts to foster learner growth and development. Two prevailing theoretical perspectives are briefly explored in the following paragraphs and presuppose that the nature of the interaction between a student and the environment impacts his or her development.

Identity development theories include personal identity theories, sociocultural identity theories, and career development theories. These theoretical frameworks focus on how our learners come to know themselves personally, interpersonally, professionally, and culturally, as well as how they come to know and understand their values, their personal and professional purpose, and their relationships. These theories posit that the better one understands oneself and one's purpose, the more comfortable one becomes moving across cultural boundaries to interact with and understand others (Broido & Schreiber, 2016).

Alternatively, *cognitive-structural development* theories attempt to explain how students learn increasingly complex forms of reasoning. These theories postulate that when the known is no longer sufficient to explain an experience, cognitive disequilibrium ensues, forcing the student to consider new alternatives and explanations (Broido & Schreiber, 2016). However, understanding of student development continues to evolve (Jones & Stewart, 2016), and scholars more recently are considering critical and poststructural theories that challenge the earlier constructs. Because nursing education is a microcosm of the higher education environment, nurse educators are encouraged to explore various theories of student development as they plan curricula and other programmatic aspects of nursing education.

Working with Diverse Learners

Postsecondary educators are called upon to facilitate learning for an increasingly diverse student body. According to the National Center for Education Statistics (2016), college enrollment is projected to set new records through fall 2025. Moreover, the demographic makeup of the undergraduate student body has evolved over time. For example, in 2015, Caucasian students accounted for 56.5 percent of students, down from 83.4 percent in 1976. During the same time frame, the percentage of black and Hispanic students more than doubled, having gone from 26.8 percent to 57.5 percent. These demographic changes are projected to continue, and by 2050 the general student body will likely be a minority majority (Chun & Evans, 2016).

Although less diverse than the general collegiate student body, trends toward a more diverse student body within nursing education are evident, and our students are more diverse than faculty. As of 2014, the National League for Nursing (NLN) reported increases in black (12.2 percent), Hispanic (8.1 percent), and Asian or Pacific Islander (5.9 percent) students, up from 9.4 percent, 3.5 percent, and 4.0 percent, respectively, in 1995. Depending on the program type, 18 percent to 42 percent of students are over the age of 30, and men account for 9 percent to 15 percent of the undergraduate and graduate student bodies.

There are multiple perspectives from which learner diversity may be considered, and each student is diverse in multiple ways. Three student subgroups are discussed in the following paragraphs, but faculty should strive to create inclusive environments where all students are respected and valued for their individual uniqueness.

English as an Additional Language Students

Language difficulties experienced by English as an additional language (EAL) students, also known as English-language learners (ELs), may be compounded in a nursing curriculum because of additional challenges associated with learning new medical terminology or communicating with staff and patients in the clinical setting. In a critical review of 25 publications, 18 of which were mostly qualitative research studies, Olson (2012) concluded that, compared to native speakers, EAL students often have higher attrition rates and lower NCLEX pass rates.

Mulready-Shick (2013) conducted a qualitative study to explore the nursing classroom experiences of 13 students from five countries. Participants reported that learning English along with the novel language of health care was even more time consuming, required adjustments in their approach to learning, and was accompanied by concerns that language difficulties would be perceived as a lack of intelligence. Along with feelings of doubt, embarrassment, and awkwardness when speaking in class, students had a strong sense of determination and focus on longer term goals. Lastly, findings from a cross-sectional, descriptive study of second-degree students in an accelerated BSN program ($n = 82$) suggest that EAL students may have difficulty with time management and control of the study environment (El-Banna, Tebbenhoff, Whitlow, & Wyche, 2017).

To assist EAL students in overcoming some of these challenges, it may be helpful to place students in study groups with speakers of the native program language, which has been shown to facilitate language skills in EAL students (Olson, 2012). In addition to language barriers, some EAL students may experience cultural conflicts with the educational or social system, while others may experience stereotyping or acts of racism by others. Thus, a climate of openness, value, and respect should be cultivated (Olson, 2012).

Veterans

Post-9/11 veterans make up approximately 4 percent of the higher education student population. Twenty percent of these major in a STEM field, while 42 percent work full time while in college (American Council on Education, 2015). Experts suggest that student veterans have many of the same issues as other adult learners, but may also have additional unique issues as a result of military service, for example, physical or psychological injury (Harborth, 2015). A growing number of researchers have begun to examine the prevalence of student veterans' mental health issues in particular. For example, when compared to nonveteran students ($n = 554$) in one statewide study, student veterans ($n = 211$) had higher prevalence of probable depression, probable posttraumatic stress disorder (PTSD), and suicide ideation. They also had a higher perceived need for treatment accompanied by higher levels of perceived stigma (Fortney et al., 2016). In a national study of student veterans ($n = 706$), respondents reported using student mental health services (89 percent), feeling mentally exhausted (71 percent), feeling overwhelmed (46 percent), and feeling lonely (43 percent); certain of these were more frequent in those deployed for hazardous duty (Albright, Fletcher, Pelts, & Taliaferro, 2017).

Research is beginning to be published in other disciplines exploring interventions to meet the needs of this student cohort. However, though some literature exists describing the development of institution-specific curricula or support services for veteran nursing students, no empirical evidence could be located specific to veterans in nursing programs.

LGBTQ Students

It is estimated that 1 million LGBTQ students are on college campuses (Tramell, 2014). Results from the Campus Pride 2010 National College Climate Survey suggest that these students are more likely than others to experience harassment, discrimination, and other forms of conduct that interfere with learning (Rankin, Weber, Blumenfeld, & Frazer, 2010), which may place these students at greater risk for mental health issues and suicide. Faculty are encouraged to become more informed about the unique needs of this student subgroup and can be a source of formal and informal support for LGBTQ students by confronting homophobic bias in the classroom, using inclusive language and preferred pronouns, and shaping course content beyond the normative curriculum to include fully representative examples (Linley et al., 2016; Rankin et al., 2010).

Accelerated BSN Students

As of June 2017, the American Association of Colleges of Nursing (AACN) listed 274 accelerated nursing programs in its directory. Students in accelerated BSN (ABSN) programs tend to have diverse characteristics, particularly as they relate to professional and life experiences (Siler, DeBasio, & Roberts, 2008). Although originally anticipated to be a collectively older student group, the average age of this cohort is consistent with the millennial generation (Bowie & Carr, 2013). Heavy academic workload in addition to family responsibilities has been identified as a major stressor for this group of students (Weitzel & McCahon, 2008). Intrinsic goal motivation may be higher for older accelerated students, while extrinsic motivation is more evident in younger accelerated students (El-Banna et al., 2017).

Academic Advising

Academic advising is viewed by many in higher education as central to both academic success and student retention efforts (Allen & Smith, 2008; White, 2015). According to the National Academic Advising Association (NACADA) (2006):

> Academic advising is integral to fulfilling the teaching and learning mission of higher education. Through academic advising, students learn to become members of their higher education community, to think critically about their roles and responsibilities as students, and to prepare to be educated citizens. (Retrieved from https://www.nacada.ksu.edu/Resources/Pillars/Concept.aspx)

Multiple philosophical frameworks from the higher education and student development literature exist to guide academic advising (Harrison, 2009a). For example, prescriptive or transactional approaches to advising focus on the mechanics of education, that is, ensuring that students enroll in appropriate courses, counseling about career options, and providing general program or organizational information. However, others view advising as a more broad-reaching, holistic, and developmental function, whereby students are guided to become lifelong learners and contemplate personal and professional success (Harrison, 2009a; Read, Hicks, & Christenbery, 2017). Particularly as the collegiate student body has diversified, the role of the adviser has expanded to focus not only on academic success but also on students' social, moral, and economic development. Thus, the role requires a unique skill set (Harborth, 2015).

Unfortunately, little attention has been given to academic advising in the nursing literature, and there is inconsistent application of the advising role, especially at the departmental and individual levels of responsibility. However, the most frequent reasons for meeting with nursing students were identified by faculty advisers in one statewide study as assisting with course registration, discussing program of study, and responding to academic difficulties or clinical difficulties (O'Neal, Zomorodi, & Wagner, 2015).

Harrison (2009a, 2009b, 2009c) conducted an extensive literature review prior to completing multiple small, single-site, descriptive studies of student and faculty perceptions of the characteristics of effective advisers in nursing education. These characteristics include being knowledgeable, available, organized, approachable, and accountable. Additionally, the most effective advisers were identified to be authentic, fostering, and nurturing advocates for their advisees and have excellent communication skills. However, faculty have reported that multiple demands on their schedule negatively impact the amount of time they are able to spend on advising and that important information, especially about educational advancement, is not always readily available (O'Neal et al., 2015).

DeLaRosby (2017) used multiple regression analysis to explore variables associated with satisfaction with academic advising in a mostly Caucasian (76 percent) and female (73 percent) general undergraduate student population ($n = 276$). Although no relationship was found between specific student characteristics (e.g., gender, race, or academic class) and satisfaction with advising, students' perceptions of both the quality of adviser-student interaction and the amount of adviser-student interaction were associated with overall satisfaction with advising.

Appreciative advising is a contemporary, developmental philosophical approach to advising whereby a collaborative relationship is forged between adviser and student to identify the student's strengths and goals to maximize success (He & Hutson, 2016; Read et al., 2017). Read et al. (2017) implemented appreciative advising in a baccalaureate program, which had previously no formal advising framework, and evaluated preliminary outcomes. A group of faculty was purposefully selected to follow the framework and met with first-year nursing students three times during the fall semester, developing rapport; assessing student strengths, goals, and fears; and assisting students to solve problems as issues arose during the semester. Students reported that they felt supported, and that issues were quickly identified and addressed. Additionally, students noted that study strategies conceived with the help of advisers had, in fact, proved helpful. Faculty advisers reported that they gained additional appreciation for the students' viewpoints and experiences, but also noted that appreciative advising was more time consuming than anticipated.

Ongoing research is needed to assist programs and faculty to better understand the role academic advising plays in the facilitation of learner development, socialization, and overall student success at both the undergraduate and graduate level. As program leaders and researchers take on this task, White (2015) cautions against defining academic advising as a service, because student satisfaction tends to be the focus of assessment, instead of short- and long-term learning outcomes resulting from advising interactions.

Understanding Learning Styles

Considerations related to learner development must take into account the unique learning styles and teaching needs of each student. There is a fairly large body of evidence in support of the idea that individual students identify with specific learning styles. That is, students have preferences for and respond differently to the manner in which information is presented to them, as well as the manner in which faculty engage them with the material (Pashler, McDaniel, Rohrer, & Bjork, 2008). Proponents of learning style research suggest that to foster development, an instructor should assess student learning styles and adapt teaching strategies to be as consistent as possible with student preferences.

References to Kolb's experiential learning theory (ELT) are common in the nursing and health care literature. ELT posits learning as a process whereby one must construct and reconstruct understanding as new exposures and experiences occur, and therefore are a major determinant of personal development. Ideally, the learner first has a concrete experience and, following reflective observation, is able to distill the experience into a more abstract conceptualization that may then be tested in active experimentation as new situations arise (Kolb & Kolb, 2005). However, in reality, there are tensions between the phases of the learning cycle, and preferences are developed among the four modes. Kolb's associated learning styles inventory seeks to assess where a student's preferences fall along two continuums—how he or she perceives information (concretely versus abstractly) and how the student processes information (actively experimenting versus reflectively observing; Pashler et al., 2008). Typically, learning styles are described based on where preferences fall into one of four quadrants created by the dissecting axes: diverging, assimilating, converging, and accommodating. Subsequently, the model has allowed for expansion from four potential learning styles to nine potential learning spaces to better differentiate the degree of preference a learner has along either axis (Kolb & Kolb, 2012).

There appears to have been little advancement in the learning styles literature since the original volume of this text was published. Most of the literature regarding learning styles remains cross-sectional and descriptive, attempting to identify learning preferences by discipline (e.g., nursing, medicine, dentistry) or other demographic characteristics such as gender, using ELT (e.g., D'Amore, James, & Mitchell, 2012; Suliman, 2010) or the VARK model (e.g., Prithishkumar & Michael, 2014), which identifies whether one has a sensory preference for visual learning, aural learning, learning by reading, or kinesthetic learning, as the basis. Collectively, the studies validate that learning styles and preferences within cohorts are diverse. Some isolated demographic associations have been identified within specific student cohorts, but it is unclear if these are reproducible across other cohorts. Suliman (2010) examined, but did not find, a link among learning style, emotional intelligence, and grade point average.

Importantly, in recent years several authors have questioned the utility of attempting to match teaching methods with student learning styles (e.g., An & Carr, 2017; Bretz, 2017; Chew, 2016; Rohrer & Pashler, 2012). Following an extensive review of the literature, Pashler et al. (2008), cognitive psychologists who were commissioned to perform the review, concluded that rigorous evidence is lacking to support widespread adoption of learning style assessment into general education practice. In particular, these authors found limited studies that employed research designs that adequately controlled for extraneous variables, leaving open the possibility that, in studies whose findings suggested that meshing teaching strategy with learning style led to improved outcomes, alternative explanations for the improved learning were possible. Additionally, in the few studies identified in which sound methodology existed, the results demonstrated no link between learning style, teaching style, and learning outcomes. Although the existence of learning preferences is not disputed, it is less well understood what their presence means or whether it is at all important that educators know and exploit them in the classroom (Pashler et al., 2008).

In an extensive review of the medical literature, Feeley and Biggerstaff (2015) examined the motivational influence behind one's approach to learning. They described a tripartite model whereby surface learning is motivated by fear of failure and tends to focus on rote learning. Strategic learning is motivated by a desire to be successful and tends to focus on the material one anticipates to see on exams. Lastly, deep learning is motivated by personal interest and a search for meaning and linkages. Following a review of 57 papers from six databases, these authors concluded that one's motivational approach to learning is likely more important than specific learning style in terms of academic success of medical students, and the strategic approach was identified as most highly correlated with exam success. Therefore, practically speaking, instead of attempting to meet the needs of diverse learners, it may be more fruitful to teach learners how to more effectively approach learning, emphasizing strategic and deep learning.

Facilitating Critical Thinking and Practice

Obviously, a major emphasis of learner development includes the manner by which educators facilitate cognitive, affective, and psychomotor achievement required of students. Since the original volume of this text was released, important work has been published that has influenced our collective thinking about learner development and socialization. As part of a series of studies sponsored by the Carnegie Foundation for the Advancement of Teaching examining the education of professionals in various professional disciplines, including medicine, law, engineering, and theology, Benner, Sutphen, Leonard, and Day (2010) published landmark findings about the nature of nursing education and the manner by which it is implemented. Using classroom observations, multiple web-based surveys, and interviews with faculty, individuals and small groups of students, preceptors, and administrators, the research team compared and evaluated nine schools of nursing in an examination of how students learn to "integrate knowledge, skilled know-how, and ethical comportment" (p. 10), which necessarily requires that students take varieties of abstract information and apply them in various forms into practice. The researchers concluded that (1) clinical practica provide meaningful learning experiences, especially when integrated with classroom content; (2) nursing programs are ineffective in the teaching of didactic types of coursework; and (3) nursing programs are adept in socializing students to the nursing role, a finding that will be discussed in more detail for its relevance to this chapter.

In response to their findings, Benner et al. (2010) suggested significant shifts in the way educators think about student learning. These suggested shifts included the need to (1) place new emphasis on "teaching for a sense of salience, situated cognition, and action in particular situations" (p. 82); (2) improve integration of classroom and clinical teaching; (3) emphasize clinical reasoning skills, of which critical thinking is only one aspect; and (4) emphasize professional formation over socialization and role taking. The Benner findings, then, inform the remainder of this chapter.

Faculty are charged with ensuring that students not just acquire knowledge but also are able to practically apply it in their practice. Although experts today recognize distinct differences in the definitions of critical thinking, clinical reasoning, and clinical judgment, for the sake of this chapter they are considered in parallel as overlapping outcomes of nursing education. Literature addressing how faculty best achieve these outcomes is examined next.

In a national survey of nurse educators, faculty (n = 143 following a 19.1 percent response rate) reported that they believe the development of critical thinking skills to be a developmental process and that inquisitiveness is the most important attribute related to critical thinking. These educators employed multiple teaching strategies, most frequently case scenarios, case studies, questioning, lecture, and discussion, to facilitate critical thinking (D. A. Clark, 2010). Additionally, in a single-site correlational study, faculty (n = 49) perceptions of personal and professional barriers to teaching critical thinking were associated with certain faculty characteristics, including educational level, academic rank, and years of teaching experience (Blondy, 2007).

Much evidence exists to inform our views about critical thinking and clinical judgment and, interestingly, some of this literature challenges long-held assumptions. For example, though it is typically presumed that critical thinking scores improve from the start to end of any nursing curriculum, a systematic review of 18 studies in four health care disciplines revealed less clear study results (Brudvig, Dirkes, Dutta, & Rane, 2013). Ten nursing studies were examined as part of the review, but only eight demonstrated improvements in critical thinking; only 11 of the full complement of 18 demonstrated change. Owing to design flaws, seven of the primary nursing studies were rated as low quality and the remainder as moderate quality. Thus, results must be considered with caution.

Two studies found in the literature attempted to identify factors that predict students' critical thinking scores as measured by the Health Science Reasoning Test (HSRT). Statistically significant relationships (at times weak) were found between critical thinking scores and time spent job-shadowing nurses and in participation in clubs and athletics (Mortellaro, 2015), as well as year of study and nursing-related experience (Hunter, Pitt, Croce, & Roche, 2014). Conversely, the studies identified no significant relationships among critical thinking and age, gender, grade point average, academic year, or learning style. Only 10 percent to 12 percent of the variance in critical thinking scores of each study was attributed to the factors identified, suggesting that additional factors relevant to critical thinking have not yet been discovered by researchers.

Teaching Strategies to Facilitate Critical Thinking

Nurse educators spend much time contemplating ways by which to facilitate critical thinking in nursing students, as it is considered a cornerstone to safe nursing practice. Since the first publication of this text, use of simulation, unfolding case studies, and concept mapping has become increasingly widespread. The influence of these teaching strategies on critical thinking is addressed next.

Simulation and Critical Thinking

Perhaps no teaching strategy has garnered as much interest in the past decade as high-fidelity simulation, and many studies have been produced in examination of its impact on various learner outcomes. The literature is replete with studies on simulation, and it is beyond the scope of this chapter to review even the highest quality studies individually.

Instead, results of multiple systematic reviews of the literature are summarized to most succinctly inform the reader of the effect of simulation on fostering critical thinking.

In an early systematic review of the simulation literature, Cant and Cooper (2010) reviewed 12 pieces of quantitative evidence examining the effectiveness of high-fidelity simulation as compared to other educational strategies. Although all 12 studies reported improvements in critical thinking, knowledge, and/or confidence associated with simulation, whether simulation was superior to comparative teaching strategies was less clear. More specifically, nine primary studies reported improvements in knowledge with various effect sizes (e.g., +7 percent and +10 percent on specific knowledge measures). However, only 5 of the 11 studies that specifically examined critical thinking as the outcome variable demonstrated improvement. Small, nonrepresentative samples and multiple other design flaws in the primary studies were identified that limit their overall validity.

Adib-Hajbaghery and Sharifi (2017) explored international databases for studies in which simulation was tested against standard or other alternative teaching methods for its effect on critical thinking in nursing students or nurses. Of 787 papers initially retrieved, 16 ultimately met the review criteria and underwent in-depth analysis of methodological quality. Nine studies used experimental design and seven used quasi-experimental design. Ten studies were conducted in the United States, four in Korea, and two in Hong Kong. Eleven of the studies used high-fidelity simulation (HFS) methods, and the others employed standardized patients (SPs), video simulation, or electronic interactive simulation. Additionally, the content, objectives, and dosing varied across the studies, as did the instruments used to measure critical thinking. Only 8 of the 16 studies reported that simulation had a positive impact on critical thinking compared to traditional or alternative teaching methods. Major methodological flaws identified in all but one of the primary studies, including inadequate blinding of outcome evaluators, lack of covert allocation, small sample sizes, and lack of cross-over contamination, necessarily reduce overall confidence in the primary study findings.

Citing the growing number of systematic reviews that address similar questions about simulation, Cant and Cooper (2017) conducted an umbrella systematic review to comprehensively review the published reviews and "to identify, appraise and review evidence on the impact of simulation-based education in pre-licensure nursing student settings" (p. 64). A comprehensive search of databases for reviews published from the years 2010 through 2015 was conducted and yielded 25 papers that met the inclusion criteria and were subsequently synthesized following guidelines put forth by the Joanna Briggs Institute. Thirteen of the papers were identified as systematic reviews, three of which included meta-analyses, and 12 were identified as integrative reviews; overall, the reviews captured more than 700 primary studies. Following the umbrella review, the authors concluded that simulation-based learning "benefited nursing students in terms of knowledge acquisition and critical thinking; it increased standardized critical thinking test scores, enhanced students' scores on knowledge and skills exams, and created a learning environment that contributed to greater knowledge, skills, safety, and students' confidence" (Cant & Cooper, 2017, p. 65). However, the authors caution that the reviews included for synthesis focused on various outcome variables, and, unfortunately, the primary studies included in each review often used various instruments to measure these variables, limiting the capability for pooling results to increase power.

To the contrary, in a landmark, rigorous, multisite, longitudinal study ($n = 666$), researchers found that use of high-fidelity simulation in replacement of either 25 percent or 50 percent of traditional clinical experiences for the duration of a nursing curriculum produced no significant differences in clinical competency, comprehensive nursing knowledge assessments, or NCLEX pass rates when compared to the control group. Additionally, there were no differences in clinical competency or readiness for practice at the six-week, three-month, and six-month periods following graduation (Hayden, Smiley, Alexander, Kardong-Edgren, & Jeffries, 2014). The validity of the study is enhanced by its rigorous design, which included thoughtfully designed simulations with reliable implementation and skilled debriefing by trained facilitators. Reproducibility of the results has significant implications for faculty workload, and it has been suggested that simulation time should be counted as more intensive than traditional clinical time (Kardong-Edgren, 2015).

Although research on the effects of simulation has grown exponentially since the first volume of this text was published, there are some troubling trends related to design flaws that confound its usefulness. More specifically, the reliance on small, single-site, or convenience samples; use of diverse outcome measures; and a lack of attention to the control of confounding variables weaken the validity of many simulation studies. To maximize research efforts, the most relevant outcome variables need to be identified so research efforts can become more efficiently focused. Issues related to dosing and other confounding variables, such as simulation instructor and environmental characteristics, need additional focus in the design of such studies. Serious discussions are needed about where research efforts should be spent, especially by doctoral students. It could be argued that producing more studies that have serious methodological flaws does not substantially advance the science and therefore should be avoided.

Unfolding Case Studies and Critical Thinking

Hong and Yu (2017) conducted a well-controlled, single-site clinical trial over two semesters in China to compare the effects of different forms of case studies on critical thinking. Multiepisodic cases (also referred to as unfolding cases) are thought to be more realistic in their capturing of the holistic and evolving human response to illness. Undergraduate students ($n = 122$) in a medical nursing course were randomly assigned to receive either multiepisodic nursing cases embedded into classroom lecture or single-episode cases. Lecturers were randomly assigned to one group or the other initially and then swapped between the groups at the midway point of each semester. Students in both groups received the same texts, reading lists, classroom hours, and clinical hours. Classes using unfolding cases started with an introduction to key background information about the disease process such as etiology and risk factors. In place of didactic lecture, relevant additional information about the diagnosis, treatment, and nursing management was uncovered as the case unfolded. Critical thinking was measured using the California Critical Thinking Disposition Inventory (CCTDI) and was similar for both groups at baseline. Although the critical thinking scores in both groups increased, the magnitude of the increase in the unfolding case group (25.06 points overall or 8.99 percent versus 9.36 points overall or 3.36 percent) was statistically significant in six of the seven critical thinking dimensions, suggesting that the use of unfolding case studies as a teaching strategy is promising. As the study was conducted at a single site in China, the generalizability may be limited.

Concept Mapping and Critical Thinking

Concept mapping is a learning strategy by which the relationships among relevant information are identified and described visually. It is thought that the mapping process helps students consider patient needs from a more holistic lens, integrate interdisciplinary knowledge into the care of the patient, and analyze the relationships among data to make more informed clinical decisions (Yue, Zhang, Zhang, & Jin, 2017). Following a thorough search of the literature, Yue et al. (2017) conducted a systematic review of 13 clinical trials (combined $n = 1,204$) to determine the effect of concept mapping on critical thinking skills. Three studies were performed in the United States, eight studies were performed in Asia (China and Taiwan), and two were performed in the Middle East (Iran and Turkey). Nine studies were performed on nursing students, while already licensed nurses participated in two studies. Seven studies ($n = 877$) measured critical thinking using the CCTDI; meta-analysis of these pooled data indicated a significant effect on critical thinking by concept mapping. Results were similar for studies using other instruments to measure critical thinking. However, caution should be used in the application of the results. Unfortunately, all of the primary studies had methodologic issues that put them at some risk for bias. For example, in none of the studies was there allocation concealment or blinding of the study participants or personnel, and only six reported randomization procedures.

Socialization and Professional Identity Formation

Crigger and Godfrey (2011) asserted that faculty should distinguish between the nurse professional and professional nurse. According to these authors, distinctions exist between being a professional nurse, one who meets the social expectations of the role, and the nurse professional, one who "has individual qualities and characteristics that inform and motivate him or her to make good moral choices" (p. xiv) while acting in the role. Nurse professionals intentionally integrate moral character with the values of nursing.

Professional identity has been referred to as "an individual's perception of himself or herself, who as a member of a profession, has responsibilities to society, recipients of care, other professionals, and to himself or herself" (Crigger & Godfrey, 2014, p. 377). This view of professional identity is broader than what previously has been conceived of as socialization, the *doing* of nursing in the form of following rules, standards, and codes. Professional identity instead requires living as and *being* a nurse through internalization of professional values and ongoing development of character and virtues (Crigger & Godfrey, 2014). Unfortunately, little is known about how to best facilitate professional identity formation and values acquisition in nursing students.

Researchers used the Nursing Professional Values Scale (NPVS) to examine students' ($n = 83$) perceptions of professional values changed during their education at one school. Statistically significant improvements in perceived importance of nursing values were identified during the final academic year, suggesting that nursing education positively impacts development (Kantek, Kaya, & Gezer, 2017). Results from a qualitative study suggest that nursing students are astute at recognizing how professional values are exemplified by nurses in practice and have identified these as being person centered, demonstrating kindness and caring, being in control, and being committed to learning. Students also recognized behavior that was in direct contrast to their understanding of professional values (Lyneham & Levett-Jones, 2016). In another qualitative study, researchers concluded that the influence of clinicians and role models, both positive and negative, also appears to have some influence on student development, values acquisition, behavior, and practice, and students seem able to distinguish between strong and poor role models (Felstead & Springett, 2016).

Socialization outcomes were assessed in ABSN students as part of the Second Careers and Nursing Program (SCAN) at one university. With clear strategies to assist students to transition into the accelerated program, move through the transition, and ultimately move out of the transition, the program formalized student-adviser relationships early on and provided a two-day orientation to help students make sense of the many practical challenges—including intense emotional responses—they would likely face as they changed professions. Peer mentoring models were instituted, and there was a focus on collaborative and contextualized learning throughout the program. Regular formative feedback was solicited from the students about the effectiveness of various teaching strategies, and timely modifications were made in response to student feedback. The curriculum culminated in a 10-week intensive internship and guided NCLEX-review. Socialization outcomes, which included validated measures of interpersonal communication, preprofessional clinical competence, cultural self-efficacy, and professional behaviors, were measured across four cohorts of students ($n = 72$) and revealed a statistically significant increase in scores from the start to the end of the program. Additionally, in a postgraduation survey, employers rated the graduates as highly competent in communication skills and ethical and moral decision-making (Dela Cruz, Farr, Klakovich, & Esslinger, 2013). Much more research is needed to understand how nursing values are acquired and developed over time, so that eventually interventions that facilitate professional identity formation might be conceived and tested.

Fostering Student Civility

Since the first edition of this text, student misbehavior and incivility have gained increasing attention as they relate to socialization and professional formation. Incivility in various forms (e.g., horizontal violence, disruptive behavior, and bullying) within the nursing profession and the broader health care arena has gained widespread discussion in the last 10 years. The topic is discussed here in relationship to nurse educators' responsibility to facilitate identity formation.

Incivility in nursing education has been defined as "rude or disruptive behaviors which often result in psychological or physiological distress for the people involved and if left unaddressed, may progress into threatening situations" (C. M. Clark, Farnsworth, & Landrum, 2009, p. 7). It may be conceived as a style of interpersonal interaction that "negatively impacts faculty and student well-being, weakens professional relationships, and impedes effective teaching and learning" (C. M. Clark & Kenaley, 2011, p. 158).

Following the seminal research of Lashley and de Meneses (2001), which documented the high percentage of faculty who had been yelled at by a nursing student in class (52.8 percent) or clinical setting (45.2 percent), or had been physically contacted in an objectionable, uninvited way (24.8 percent), Luparell (2004, 2007) reported the profound impact such experiences had on faculty. The literature is now replete with descriptive evidence establishing the ongoing nature of this problem in both the traditional and online nursing classroom (e.g., Altmiller, 2012; C. M. Clark, 2008; C. M. Clark & Springer, 2007; C. M. Clark, Werth, & Ahten, 2012; De Gagne, Choi, Ledbetter, Kang, & Clark, 2016; Luparell, 2007; Marchiondo, Marchiondo, & Lasiter, 2010; Rieck & Crouch, 2007). Uncivil behaviors take many forms and may be perceived differently by different people. They may include behaviors such as failure to engage, skipping class, eating or sleeping in class, using technology inappropriately, making disrespectful or sarcastic remarks, using foul language, or being argumentative (C. M. Clark, Farnsworth, & Landrum, 2009; Johnson, Claus, Goldman, & Sollitto, 2017). Faculty who are younger, less experienced, minorities, or women may experience more student incivility, and women may experience more serious incidents of incivility, according to a national study of faculty in higher education ($n = 524$) (Lampman, 2012).

Little is known about the factors that influence poor student behavior in nursing. Stress has been suggested as influencing both students and faculty as they interact (C. M. Clark, 2008; C. M. Clark, Nguyen, & Barbosa-Leiker, 2014). A sense of academic entitlement has also been linked to student noncompliance with rules, a specific type of uncivil behavior (Kopp & Finney, 2013).

Disruptive and uncivil behavior has been linked to poor patient safety outcomes in clinical practice (Institute for Safe Medication Practices [ISMP], 2013; Rosenstein & O'Daniel, 2008; The Joint Commission [TJC], 2008). The trend of bad student behavior toward faculty in nursing education is therefore troubling, not only because it has been linked to faculty dissatisfaction and turnover (Luparell, 2007; Walker, 2014), but also because it potentially portends bad behavior toward student peers, which has been shown to be deleterious to the mental health and well-being of the target (Sauer, Hannon, & Beyer, 2017), or toward health care team members in postlicensure practice.

In a national survey, 37 percent of faculty respondents ($n = 1,869$) reported that they were aware of at least one former student whom they perceived to be unprofessional or uncivil as a student who subsequently behaved unprofessionally or uncivilly as a licensed nurse (Luparell & Frisbee, 2014). Additionally, 71 percent reported thinking that at least one student who graduated in the past academic year should not have graduated because of bad behavior. An astonishing 54.7 percent indicated thinking that at least two students who graduated should not have been allowed to graduate. These findings are consistent with those of other researchers who have reported on a phenomenon referred to as "failing to fail" (Docherty & Dieckmann, 2015; Luhanga, Yonge, & Myrick, 2008).

Additional findings from the national faculty survey revealed that most faculty (96.5 percent, 73.3 percent, and 57.4 percent, respectively) believe that nursing programs have a responsibility to address uncivil student behavior, that poorly behaving students will go on to be poorly behaving licensed nurses, and that consistently uncivil students should not pass a course, even if they have earned a passing mark in traditional assessment measures.

Incivility has been likened to a dance, suggesting that both student and teacher share responsibility for the manner in which encounters unfold (C. M. Clark, 2008). Indeed, some evidence exists that instructor traits and characteristics may play mediating roles in student incivility. The relationship among instructor credibility, instructor self-disclosure (i.e., the sharing of relevant personal and professional information with students), and nonverbal immediacy to student incivility was studied in a large group of students ($n = 438$) representing more than 40 majors at a single, large university (Miller, Katt, Brown, & Sivo, 2014). Findings suggest that when an instructor is perceived by students as credible, there are lower levels of student incivility, and the nature of instructor self-disclosure was linked to instructor credibility. Thus, faculty may wish to develop their nonverbal immediacy skills (e.g., smiling, gesturing, making eye contact, using appropriate vocal inflections, and listening actively), while avoiding specific types of negative self-disclosure (e.g., personal failures and character weaknesses) that may detract from their credibility.

Unfortunately, the brunt of the academic incivility scholarship to date remains descriptive in nature, and few researchers have examined interventions to ameliorate the problem. Only recently have researchers attempted to study specific interventions to reduce student incivility. For example, Authement (2016) studied student perceptions of incivility following implementation of a faculty-developed code of conduct. A 25 percent reduction in perceived incivility was reported. Jenkins, Kerber, and Woith (2013) enlisted 10 nursing student leaders to participate in a weekly journal club emphasizing civility and team building. The student leaders were then expected to role model behaviors and skills in subsequent interactions with classmates and faculty. The students reported a change in behavior and attitudes regarding civility and the use of a wider array of coping mechanisms.

These and the few other interventional studies in the literature are important first steps, but they lack clarity and rigor. They are typically single-site studies with small, often self-selected samples, and are lacking in long-term assessment of meaningful outcomes. The educational interventions tend to be poorly defined, and there are confounding variables that are not considered, for example, teaching skill or individual characteristics of the instructor.

GAPS IN THE RESEARCH

Despite advancements in specific areas, for example, the influence of specific teaching strategies on critical thinking, there is still much we do not understand about how to best facilitate overall learner development and socialization. For example, we need to learn more about the role of both formal and informal interactions with students, by whom these should be conducted, and how these impact students' development and overall success in nursing education. Research is also needed to enhance our understanding of how to meet the needs of specific subgroups of students. Additionally, much of the literature on learner development focuses on prelicensure nursing students. As graduate students increase in number, especially in programs that prepare them to take on new roles as scholars or advanced practitioners, we need to better understand how they can best be helped to move into these new roles and to what degree the undergraduate evidence is generalizable to the graduate student population. This is an especially important consideration in the design of academic progression programs (e.g., BSN to PhD or BSN to DNP).

While innovative teaching strategies are conceived, implemented, and tested frequently in nursing programs all over the world, often they are evaluated only at the classroom or programmatic level. Few studies take into account the multiple variables that may influence successful implementation of these strategies elsewhere. For example, are there faculty traits or characteristics that impact the success of even the most well-developed intervention? Conversely, are there primary structural elements to a teaching strategy that would lead to success regardless of where and by whom it is implemented? More research needs to examine the relationship among educators, students, the environment, and teaching strategies, and how these affect student success.

Lastly, devoted effort is needed to understand how to best assist students in the complex area of socialization and professional identity formation. We know little about how students acquire nursing values, the clinical importance of such acquisition, or if there are interventions available to actively facilitate such acquisition. In terms of professional behavior and comportment, we need to better understand linkages between behavior as a student and behavior later in practice.

PRIORITIES FOR FUTURE RESEARCH

Learner development is holistic and encompasses many aspects of student growth along a continuum. Much of the research about learner development and socialization in nursing remains descriptive or has significant methodological flaws that limit its utility. To maximally advance the science, well-designed and rigorous studies are needed that answer the following questions:

> What outcomes are the most important when considering learner development, and how can they be measured?

> What are the most effective advising, counseling, or mentoring strategies to assist students?

> What are the unique needs of specific subgroups of students, and how can these needs best be met?

> What teacher, student, or environmental characteristics influence the success of a teaching strategy?

> How can professional identity formation be measured?

> What are the predictive factors for professional identity formation?

> What student, teacher, and program factors contribute to or predict student incivility?

> Which, if any, student behaviors or characteristics predict postlicensure behavior and practice?

> How should student behavior be evaluated and to what end?

> What interventions are effective to facilitate professional values acquisition or create long-term change in professional comportment?

References

Adib-Hajbaghery, M., & Sharifi, N. (2017). Effect of simulation training on the development of nurses and nursing students' critical thinking: A systematic literature review. *Nurse Education Today*, *50*(Suppl, C), 17–24. doi:10.1016/j.nedt.2016.12.011

Albright, D. L., Fletcher, K. L., Pelts, M. D., & Taliaferro, L. (2017). Use of college mental health services among student veterans. *Best Practice in Mental Health*, *13*(1), 65–79.

Allen, J. M., & Smith, C. L. (2008). Importance of, responsibility for, and satisfaction with academic advising: A faculty perspective. *Journal of College Student Development*, *49*(5), 397–411. doi:10.1353/csd.0.0033

Altmiller, G. (2012). Student perceptions of incivility in nursing education: Implications for educators. *Nursing Education Perspectives*, *33*(1), 15–20. doi:10.5480/1536-5026-33.1.15

An, D., & Carr, M. (2017). Learning styles theory fails to explain learning and achievement: Recommendations for alternative approaches. *Personality & Individual Differences*, *116*, 410–416. doi:10.1016/j.paid.2017.04.050

American Association of Colleges of Nursing. (2017). *Nursing education programs*. Retrieved December 2, 2017, from http://www.aacnnursing.org/Nursing-Education

American Council on Education (ACE). (2015, Spring). *By the numbers: Undergraduate student veterans*. Retrieved from http://www.acenet.edu/the-presidency/columns-and-features/Pages/By-the-Numbers-Undergraduate-Student-Veterans.aspx

Authement, R. (2016). Incivility in nursing students. *Nursing Management*, *47*(11), 36–43. doi:10.1097/01.NUMA.0000497005.19670.9f

Benner, P., Sutphen, M., Leonard, V., & Day, L. (2010). *Educating nurses: A call for radical transformation*. San Francisco, CA: Jossey-Bass.

Blondy, L. C. (2007). *A correlational study between the critical thinking skills of nursing faculty and their perceived barriers to teaching critical thinking skills to nursing*

students (Order No. 3288871). Available from ProQuest Central; ProQuest Dissertations & Theses Global. (304720478). Retrieved from https://search.proquest.com/docview/304720478?accountid=28148

Bowie, B. H., & Carr, K. C. (2013). From coach to colleague: Adjusting pedagogical approaches and attitudes in accelerated nursing programs. *Journal of Professional Nursing*, *29*(6), 395–401. doi:10.1016/j.profnurs.2012.05.016

Bretz, S. L. (2017). Finding no evidence for learning styles. *Journal of Chemical Education*, *94*(7), 825–826. doi:10.1021/acs.jchemed.7b00424

Broido, E. M., & Schreiber, B. (2016). Promoting student learning and development. *New Directions for Higher Education*, *2016*(175), 65–74. doi:10.1002/he.20200

Brudvig, T. J., Dirkes, A., Dutta, P., & Rane, K. (2013). Critical thinking skills in health care professional students: A systematic review. *Journal of Physical Therapy Education*, *27*(3), 12–25.

Cant, R. P., & Cooper, S. J. (2010). Simulation-based learning in nurse education: Systematic review. *Journal of Advanced Nursing*, *66*(1), 3–15. doi:10.1111/j.1365-2648.2009.05240.x

Cant, R. P., & Cooper, S. J. (2017). Use of simulation-based learning in undergraduate nurse education: An umbrella systematic review. *Nurse Education Today*, *49*, 63–71. doi:10.1016/j.nedt.2016.11.015

Chew, K. S. (2016). Tailoring teaching instructions according to student's different learning styles: Are we hitting the right button? *Education in Medicine Journal*, *8*(3), 103–107. doi:10.5959/eimj.v8i3.455

Chun, E., & Evans, A. (2016). Rethinking cultural competence in higher education: An ecological framework for student development. *ASHE Higher Education Report*, *42*(4), 7–162. doi:10.1002/aehe.20102

Clark, C. M. (2008). The dance of incivility in nursing education as described by nursing faculty and students. *Advances in Nursing Science, 31*(4), e37.

Clark, C. M., Farnsworth, J., & Landrum, R. E. (2009). Development and description of the Incivility in Nursing Education (INE) Survey. *Journal of Theory Construction & Testing, 13*(1), 7–15.

Clark, C. M., & Kenaley, B. L. (2011). Faculty empowerment of students to foster civility in nursing education: A merging of two conceptual models. *Nursing Outlook, 59*(3), 158. doi:10.1016/j.outlook.2010.12.005

Clark, C. M., Nguyen, D. T., & Barbosa-Leiker, C. (2014). Student perceptions of stress, coping, relationships, and academic civility: A longitudinal study. *Nurse Educator, 39*(4), 170–174. doi:10.1097/NME.0000000000000049

Clark, C. M., & Springer, P. (2007). Incivility in nursing education: A descriptive study on definitions and prevalence. *Journal of Nursing Education, 46*(1), 7–14.

Clark, C. M., Werth, L., & Ahten, S. (2012). Cyber-bullying and incivility in the online learning environment, part 1: Addressing faculty and student perceptions. *Nurse Educator, 37*(4), 150–156. doi:10.1097/NNE.0b013e31825a87e5

Clark, D. A. (2010). *Nursing faculty perceptions on teaching critical thinking* (Doctoral dissertation, Capella University). Retrieved from http://search.ebscohost.com.proxybz.lib. montana.edu/login.aspx?direct=true&db=ccm&AN=109853459&login.asp&site=ehost-live

Crigger, N., & Godfrey, N. (2011). *The making of nurse professionals: A transformational, ethical approach.* Sudbury, MA: Jones & Bartlett Learning.

Crigger, N., & Godfrey, N. (2014). From the inside out: A new approach to teaching professional identity formation and professional ethics. *Journal of Professional Nursing, 30*(5), 376–382. doi:10.1016/j.profnurs.2014.03.004

D'Amore, A., James, S., & Mitchell, E. K. L. (2012). Learning styles of first-year undergraduate nursing and midwifery students: A cross-sectional survey utilising the Kolb Learning Style Inventory. *Nurse Education Today, 32*(5), 506–515. doi:10.1016/j.nedt.2011.08.001

De Gagne, J. C., Choi, M., Ledbetter, L., Kang, H. S., & Clark, C. M. (2016). An integrative review of cybercivility in health professions education. *Nurse Educator, 41*(5), 239–245. doi:10.1097/nne.0000000000000264

Dela Cruz, F. A., Farr, S., Klakovich, M. D., & Esslinger, P. (2013). Facilitating the career transition of second-career students into professional nursing. *Nursing Education Perspectives, 34*(1), 12–17. doi:10.5480%2F1536-5026-34.1.12

DeLaRosby, H. R. (2017). Student characteristics and collegiate environments that contribute to the overall satisfaction with academic advising among college students. *Journal of College Student Retention: Research, Theory & Practice, 19*(2), 145–160. doi:10.1353/jge.2015.0024

Docherty, A., & Dieckmann, N. (2015). Is there evidence of failing to fail in our schools of nursing? *Nursing Education Perspectives, 36*(4), 226–231. doi:10.5480/14-1485

El-Banna, M. M., Tebbenhoff, B., Whitlow, M., & Wyche, K. F. (2017). Motivated strategies for learning in accelerated second-degree nursing students. *Nurse Educator, 42*(6), 308–312. doi:10.1097/NNE.0000000000000391

Feeley, A.-M., & Biggerstaff, D. L. (2015). Exam success at undergraduate and graduate-entry medical schools: Is learning style or learning approach more important? A critical review exploring links between academic success, learning styles, and learning approaches among school-leaver entry ("traditional") and graduate-entry ("nontraditional") medical students. *Teaching & Learning in Medicine, 27*(3), 237–244. doi:10.1080/10401334.2015.1046734

Felstead, I. S., & Springett, K. (2016). An exploration of role model influence on adult nursing students' professional development: A phenomenological research study. *Nurse Education Today, 37*, 66–70. doi:10.1016/j.nedt.2015.11.014

Fortney, J. C., Curran, G. M., Hunt, J. B., Cheney, A. M., Lu, L., Valenstein, M., & Eisenberg, D. (2016). Prevalence of probable mental disorders and help-seeking behaviors among veteran and non-veteran community college students. *General Hospital Psychiatry, 38*, 99–104. doi:10.1016/j.genhosppsych.2015.09.007

Harborth, A. (2015). The developing role of student advising: An interview with Charlie Nutt. *Journal of Developmental Education, 39*(1), 18–20.

Harrison, E. (2009a). (Re)visiting academic advising. *Nurse Educator, 34*(2), 64–68. doi:10.1097/NNE.0b013e31819907ff

Harrison, E. (2009b). Faculty perceptions of academic advising: "I don't get no respect." *Nursing Education Perspectives, 30*(4), 229–233. doi:10.1016/S0168-8510(09)70006-5

Harrison, E. (2009c). What constitutes good academic advising? Nursing students' perceptions of academic advising. *Journal of Nursing Education, 48*(7), 361–366. doi:10.3928/01484834-20090615-02

Hayden, J., Smiley, R. A., Alexander, M., Kardong-Edgren, S., & Jeffries, P. (2014). The NCSBN National Simulation Study. *Journal of Nursing Regulation, 5*(2 Suppl.), S3-S64. doi:10.1016/j.ecns.2012.07.070

He, Y., & Hutson, B. (2016). Appreciative assessment in academic advising. *Review of Higher Education, 39*(2), 213–240. doi:10.1353/rhe.2016.0003

Hong, S., & Yu, P. (2017). Comparison of the effectiveness of two styles of case-based learning implemented in lectures for developing nursing students' critical thinking ability: A randomized controlled trial. *International Journal of Nursing Studies, 68*, 16–24. doi:10.1016/j.ijnurstu.2016.12.008

Hunter, S., Pitt, V., Croce, N., & Roche, J. (2014). Critical thinking skills of undergraduate nursing students: Description and demographic predictors. *Nurse Education Today, 34*(5), 809–814. doi:10.1016/j.nedt.2013.08.005

Institute for Safe Medication Practices (ISMP). (2013). Unresolved disrespectful behavior in healthcare: Practitioners speak up (again), part 1. *ISMP Safety Alert Newsletter/Nurse Advise-ERR, 11*(10), 1–4.

Jenkins, S. D., Kerber, C. S., & Woith, W. M. (2013). An intervention to promote civility among nursing students. *Nursing Education Perspectives, 34*(2), 95–100.

Johnson, Z. D., Claus, C. J., Goldman, Z. W., & Sollitto, M. (2017). College student misbehaviors: An exploration of instructor perceptions. *Communication Education, 66*(1), 54–69. doi:10.1080/03634523.2016.1202995

The Joint Commission. (2008). *Sentinel event alert 40: Behaviors that undermine a culture of safety*. Retrieved from http://www.joint-commission.org/assets/1/18/SEA_40.PDF

Jones, S. R., & Stewart, D. L. (2016). Evolution of student development theory. *New Directions for Student Services, 2016*(154), 17–28. doi:10.1002/ss.20172

Kantek, F., Kaya, A., & Gezer, N. (2017). The effects of nursing education on professional values: A longitudinal study. *Nurse Education Today, 58*, 43–46. doi:10.1016/j.nedt.2017.08.004

Kardong-Edgren, S. (2015). Initial thoughts after the NCSBN National Simulation Study. *Clinical Simulation in Nursing, 11*(4), 201–202. doi:10.1016/j.ecns.2015.02.005

Kolb, A. Y., & Kolb, D. A. (2005). Learning styles and learning spaces: Enhancing experiential learning in higher education. *Academy of Management Learning and Education, 4*(2), 193–212.

Kolb, A. Y., & Kolb, D. A. (2012). Experiential learning spaces. In N. M. Seel (Eds.), *Encyclopedia of the sciences of learning*. Boston, MA: Springer. doi:10.1007/978-1-4419-1428-6

Kopp, J. P., & Finney, S. J. (2013). Linking academic entitlement and student incivility using latent means modeling. *Journal of Experimental Education, 81*(3), 322–336. doi:10.1080/00220973.2012.727887

Lampman, C. (2012). Women faculty at risk: U.S. professors report on their experiences with student incivility, bullying, aggression, and sexual attention. *NASPA Journal About Women in Higher Education, 5*(2), 184–208. doi:https://doi.org/10.1515/njawhe-2012-1108

Lashley, F. R., & de Meneses, M. (2001). Student civility in nursing programs: A national survey. *Journal of Professional Nursing, 17*(2), 81–86. doi:10.1053/jpnu.2001.22271

Linley, J. L., Nguyen, D., Brazelton, G. B., Becker, B., Renn, K., & Woodford, M. (2016). Faculty as sources of support for LGBTQ college students. *College Teaching, 64*(2), 55–63. doi:10.1080/87567555.2015.1078275

Luhanga, F., Yonge, O. J., & Myrick, F. (2008). "Failure to assign failing grades": Issues with grading the unsafe student. *International Journal of Nursing Education Scholarship, 5*(1), Article 8.

Luparell, S. (2004). Faculty encounters with uncivil nursing students: an overview. *Journal of Professional Nursing, 20*(1), 59–67.

Luparell, S. (2007). The effects of student incivility on nursing faculty. *Journal of Nursing Education, 46*(1), 15–19.

Luparell, S., & Frisbee, K. (2014). *Do uncivil nursing students become uncivil nurses?* Paper presented at the National League for Nursing Education Summit, Phoenix, AZ.

Lyneham, J., & Levett-Jones, T. (2016). Insights into registered nurses' professional values through the eyes of graduating students. *Nurse Education in Practice, 17*, 86–90. doi:10.1016/j.nepr.2015.11.002

Marchiondo, K., Marchiondo, L. A., & Lasiter, S. (2010). Faculty incivility: Effects on program satisfaction of BSN students. *Journal of Nursing Education, 49*(11), 608.

Miller, A. N., Katt, J. A., Brown, T., & Sivo, S. A. (2014). The relationship of instructor self-disclosure, nonverbal immediacy, and credibility to student incivility in the college classroom. *Communication Education, 63*(1), 1–16. doi:10.1080/03634523.2013.835054

Mortellaro, C. (2015). *Exploring factors influencing critical thinking skills in undergraduate nursing students: A mixed methods study* (Order No. 3729603). Available from ProQuest Dissertations & Theses Global. (1731113650). Retrieved from https://search.proquest.com/docview/1731113650?accountid=28148

Mulready-Shick, J. (2013). A critical exploration of how English language learners experience nursing education. *Nursing Education Perspectives (National League for Nursing), 34*(2), 82–87. doi:10.5480/1536-5026-34.2.82

National Academic Advising Association (NACADA): The Global Community for Academic Advising. (2006). *NACADA concept of academic advising*. Retrieved from NACADA Clearinghouse of Academic Advising Resources website: http://www.nacada.ksu.edu/Resources/Clearinghouse/View-Articles/Concept-of-Academic-Advising-a598.aspx

National Center for Education Statistics. (2016, October). Higher Education General Information Survey (HEGIS), "Fall Enrollment in Colleges and Universities" surveys, 1976 and 1980; Integrated Postsecondary Education Data System (IPEDS), "Fall Enrollment Survey" (IPEDS-EF:90); and IPEDS Spring 2001 through Spring 2016, Fall Enrollment component. Washington, DC: US Department of Education.

National League for Nursing. (2014). Nursing student demographics. Retrieved from http://www.nln.org/newsroom/nursing-education-statistics/nursing-student-demographics

Olson, M. (2012). English-as-a-second language (ESL) nursing student success: A critical review of the literature. *Journal of Cultural Diversity, 19*(1), 26–32.

O'Neal, D., Zomorodi, M., & Wagner, J. (2015). Nursing education progression. *Nurse Educator, 40*(3), 129–133. doi:10.1097/NNE.0000000000000128

Owen, J. E. (2012). Using student development theories as conceptual frameworks in leadership education. *New Directions for Student Services, 2012*(140), 17–35. doi:10.1002/ss.20029

Pashler, H., McDaniel, M., Rohrer, D., & Bjork, R. (2008). Learning styles: Concepts and evidence. *Psychological Science in the Public Interest, 9*(3), 105–119. doi:10.1111/j.1539-6053.2009.01038.x

Patton, L. D., Renn, K. A., Guido, F. M., & Quaye, S. J. (2016). *Student development in college: Theory, research, and practice* (3rd ed.). San Francisco, CA: Jossey-Bass.

Prithishkumar, I., & Michael, S. (2014). Understanding your student: Using the VARK model. *Journal of Postgraduate Medicine, 60*(2), 183–186.

Rankin, S., Weber, G., Blumenfeld, W., & Frazer, S. (2010). *2010 state of higher education for lesbian, gay, bisexual & transgender people.* Charlotte, NC: Campus Pride.

Read, A., Hicks, J., & Christenbery, T. (2017). Appreciative advising in nursing education. *Nurse Educator, 42*(2), 81–84. doi:10.1097/NNE.0000000000000304

Rieck, S., & Crouch, L. (2007). Connectiveness and civility in online learning. *Nurse Education in Practice, 7*(6), 425.

Rohrer, D., & Pashler, H. (2012). Learning styles: Where's the evidence? *Medical Education, 46*(7), 634–635. doi:10.1111/j.1365-2923.2012.04273.x

Rosenstein, A. H., & O'Daniel, M. (2008). A survey of the impact of disruptive behaviors and communication defects on patient safety. *Joint Commission Journal on Quality and Patient Safety/Joint Commission Resources, 34*(8), 464–471.

Sauer, P. A., Hannon, A. E., & Beyer, K. B. (2017). Peer incivility among prelicensure nursing students: A call to action for nursing faculty. *Nurse Educator, 42*(6), 281–285. doi:10.1097/NNE.0000000000000375

Siler, B., DeBasio, N., & Roberts, K. (2008). Profile of non-nurse college graduates enrolled in accelerated baccalaureate curricula: Results of a national study. *Nursing Education Perspectives, 29*(6), 336–341.

Suliman, W. A. (2010). The relationship between learning styles, emotional social intelligence, and academic success of undergraduate nursing students. *Journal of Nursing Research, 18*(2), 136–143.

Tramell, J. B. (2014, May/June). LGBT challenges in higher education: 5 core principles for success. Retrieved from https://www.agb.org/trusteeship/2014/5/lgbt-challenges-higher-education-today-5-core-principles-success

Walker, R. Y. (2014). *Incivility in nursing education: Its effect on the job satisfaction of nurse faculty in associate degree programs* (Order No. 3629352). Available from ProQuest Dissertations & Theses Global. (1564222097). Retrieved from https://search.proquest.com/docview/1564222097?accountid=28148

Weitzel, M. L., & McCahon, C. P. (2008). Stressors and supports for baccalaureate nursing students completing an accelerated program. *Journal of Professional Nursing, 24*(2), 85–89.

White, E. R. (2015). Academic advising in higher education: A place at the core. *Journal of General Education, 64*(4), 263–277.

Yue, M., Zhang, M., Zhang, C., & Jin, C. (2017). The effectiveness of concept mapping on development of critical thinking in nursing education: A systematic review and meta-analysis. *Nurse Education Today, 52*, 87–94. doi:10.1016/j.nedt.2017.02.018

5

Competency III: Use Assessment and Evaluation Strategies

Darrell Spurlock, Jr., PhD, RN, NEA-BC, ANEF

Bette Mariani, PhD, RN, ANEF

Assessment and evaluation of student learning, especially those assessment and evaluation activities carried out at the level of individual students and groups of students involved in classroom, clinical, and laboratory learning contexts, are among the most important and consequential educational activities for both students and nurse educators alike. The National League for Nursing *Scope of Practice for Academic Nurse Educators©* (NLN, 2012c) outlines the essential knowledge, skills, and abilities required for nurse educators to effectively use assessment and evaluation strategies in *Competency III: Use Assessment and Evaluation Strategies,* which specifies that to use assessment and evaluation strategies effectively, the nurse educator

> ▸ uses extant literature to develop evidence-based assessment and evaluation practices;
>
> ▸ uses a variety of strategies to assess and evaluate learning in the cognitive, psychomotor, and affective domains;
>
> ▸ implements evidence-based assessment and evaluation strategies that are appropriate to the learner and to learning goals;
>
> ▸ uses assessment and evaluation data to enhance the teaching/learning process;
>
> ▸ provides timely, constructive, and thoughtful feedback to learners; and
>
> ▸ demonstrates skill in the design and use of tools for assessing clinical practice.

Because nurse educators hold primary responsibility for assessing and evaluating nursing students' learning and skills in a variety of contexts and settings—and in a variety of domains (cognitive, psychomotor, and affective)—they must be versed in a wide variety of assessment and evaluation techniques. These include, but are not limited to, test item writing and analysis of classroom exams; selection and interpretation of standardized, commercially available exams; and clinical and laboratory skill performance evaluation. Nurse educators are also responsible for the evaluation of nonclinical student learning outcomes including students' professional writing skills and abilities; development of professional values, beliefs, and attitudes; and interpersonal and social capabilities, such as those required for effective teamwork; communication with patients, families, and colleagues; and leadership skills. Just as the NLN (2012c) has noted, while individual nurse educators are not expected to demonstrate expertise across all these domains and methods of assessment, the nursing faculty as a whole should possess sufficient expertise in all the required assessment and evaluation competency areas to ensure that students receive a robust, evidence-based assessment and evaluation experience within their programs.

REVIEW OF THE LITERATURE

The evidence base supporting nurse educator competence in assessment and evaluation strategies is complicated and, especially regarding nursing-education-specific assessment and evaluation strategies, highly underdeveloped. The underdeveloped nature of the nursing education measurement and assessment literature was identified in Halstead (2007), which represented the first published literature review related to the nurse educator core competencies. Unfortunately, this critical limitation continues (Ironside & Spurlock, 2014; Tanner, 2011).

To illustrate the limited literature base available, a search of Cumulative Index to Nursing and Allied Health Literature (CINAHL), using the MeSH heading and subheading for MH "Education, Nursing Evaluation" for entries published from 2005 to 2017, produced only 232 results, of which only a fraction were data-based manuscripts. Limiting the search further to items with a geographic coding for the United States resulted in 72 entries only.

When examining the assessment and evaluation literature as a whole, one very important consideration nurse educators must make is that assessment and evaluation practices are guided, perhaps in equal parts, by ethical/philosophical principles and frameworks, statistical and measurement theory, and empirical evidence (generally supporting validity and reliability claims). Therefore, the literature relevant to assessment and evaluation practices cannot be limited to published empirical research findings, but must also include guidelines from professional organizations, widely accepted fair testing frameworks, and theoretical literature from a diversity of fields that has grown and developed over the past nine decades of modern educational and psychometric measurement practice.

To provide readers with a solid foundation in educational assessment and evaluation practices, we refer interested readers to the following well-regarded textbooks, some of which are nursing education focused and some of which are used more generally in graduate-level education and social science programs. First, Thorndike and Thorndike-Christ (2011) provide a very accessible and interdisciplinary introduction to educational assessment and evaluation theory and research from a strongly psychological perspective. Now in its eighth edition, the Thorndike and Thorndike-Christ text provides an especially good review of content relevant to nurse educators working with large-scale, commercially available standardized nursing knowledge tests, which are common in nursing education programs today. In an equally rigorous treatment of educational assessment and evaluation content written specifically for nurse educators, McDonald (2014) provides a comprehensive reference with a strong focus on test item writing, item analysis, evaluation of clinical and laboratory learning, and preparing students for the national nursing licensure examination (NCLEX). Likewise, Oermann and Gaberson's (2014) reference text on assessment and evaluation in nursing education is comprehensive, up to date, and reflective of best practices, and should be considered an essential resource for nurse educators or nursing education students at any level.

For nurse educators interested in an authoritative reference specifically focused on the technical and empirical underpinnings of educational test development and evaluation, with a focus on large-scale assessment, administration, and scoring and good coverage of classroom test development, Lane, Raymond, and Haladyna (2016) have assembled a gold standard reference work dedicated to that purpose. Lastly, readers interested in a robust but accessible nontest, psychometric scale development and evaluation reference are referred to DeVellis (2016), who provides an excellent discussion and introduction to validity and reliability theory and, of course, a thorough guide to developing and testing new psychometric scales, such as those used to measure attitudes, beliefs, values, and other latent constructs—which are often of interest to nurse educators.

Several key guidelines and frameworks from professional organizations also serve as influential resources in any discussion of educational assessment and evaluation. First, the *Standards for Educational and Psychological Testing* are gold standard testing guidelines jointly published by the American Education Research Association (AERA), the American Psychological Association (APA), and the National Council on Measurement in Education (NCME). First published in 1966, the standards (AERA, APA, & NCME, 2014) reflect the collective professional expertise of testing and assessment practitioners and researchers from three of the top national professional organizations dedicated to rigorous, evidence-based, fair testing practices across all types of educational and occupational settings in the United States.

Providing discipline-specific guidance to nurse educators, the NLN (2012b) described the challenges and opportunities nurse educators face when using commercially available standardized nursing content exams in high-stakes situations. The NLN also published a set of fair testing guidelines (NLN, 2012a), which outlines steps nurse educators should take when selecting, implementing, and evaluating commercially available standardized examinations, with special consideration for how these exams should be used when important educational decisions, such as whether students will progress in or graduate from a nursing education program, are made based on students' test scores.

To supplement the authoritative resources described previously with the most recent empirical and theoretical findings within the field of nursing education, the CINAHL, Education Resources Information Center (ERIC), PsychINFO, MEDLINE, and several commercially organized EBSCOhost education and social-science-oriented literature databases were searched for nursing-education-specific assessment and evaluation papers published from 2005 through early 2017. Searches generally excluded items published outside academic journals (e.g., dissertations) and papers originating outside the United States, with rare exceptions. Additionally, papers reporting findings from small ($N < 50$) single-site studies, pilot studies, or quality improvement projects were omitted from substantive consideration, and reprints of papers published prior to 2005 were excluded.

The literature database searches revealed a few themes in nursing education literature over the last decade, including high-stakes testing in both classroom and laboratory/

simulation settings, development of clinical judgment models and associated rubrics to evaluate student clinical learning and performance, and, finally, a limited expansion of scholarship on assessment and evaluation of student learning outcomes peripheral to content knowledge, such as those related to critical thinking, professional values and attitudes, and teamwork skills. These themes reflect, in part, a literature dominated by a focus on undergraduate, prelicensure students with very little attention paid to graduate nursing education. Lastly, selected highly cited or otherwise influential papers from the fields of education, educational psychology, and other health professions are included throughout the chapter to further supplement assessment and evaluation practice competencies relevant to nurse educators. Readers will see the themes and topics previously outlined addressed throughout the chapter under the familiar headings of assessment and evaluation in the cognitive, affective, and psychomotor domains, as appropriate.

Key Definitions

To situate the reader within the sometimes specialized language of assessment and evaluation, several key definitions are provided here. These definitions are generally considered to be widely accepted—but because no definitive standard definitions exist, some variability across sources and fields of study is entirely expected. First, though the terms *assessment* and *evaluation* are often used interchangeably, for the purposes of this chapter and consistent with definitions provided by McDonald (2014), Oermann and Gaberson (2014), and Thorndike and Thorndike-Christ (2011), assessment is defined as the process by which nurse educators gather and collect data about student knowledge, skills, and abilities to make educational decisions. Central to gathering assessment data is the act of *measurement*, defined as the assigning of numerical values or scores to represent the amount of the underlying construct or trait being measured; the most common construct of interest to nurse educators, and educators of all types, is knowledge.

Once measurement data have been collected through the assessment process, making educational decisions based on that data is the formal definition of *evaluation*, which, as McDonald (2014) notes, involves assigning meaning (or value) to the assessment data, usually in light of predefined performance or achievement standards. The clearest illustration of the act of evaluation is in the assigning of grades: student-level assessment data are collected through a variety of methods across the course of a semester and at the conclusion of the course; those data are evaluated in sum to assign the student a final course grade. In this common scenario, the faculty member (or the faculty as a whole) has predetermined the performance and achievement levels necessary to pass or fail the course and, to provide an even finer level of detail, have established more discrete categories to classify a student's level of achievement (e.g., A+, B, C-, etc.).

Another common and well-accepted nomenclature involves the terms *formative* and *summative*, usually paired with the word *assessment* (e.g., *formative assessment, summative assessment*). Formative assessment involves measuring and providing direct feedback on student learning or performance with the intended goal of helping the student improve prior to the summative, or evaluation, stage. Formative assessment is primarily viewed as an instructional strategy or method. Summative assessment involves making a judgment about the level of achievement, performance, or mastery that a student demonstrates. Because formative assessment is primarily focused on promoting learning (rather than rendering judgments), the focus in this chapter is on the summative, or primarily evaluative, aspects of assessment.

Validity and Reliability in Educational Contexts

A theme throughout this chapter—and indeed throughout most of the assessment and evaluation literature—is the central importance of two educational measurement concepts: *validity* and *reliability*. A major development since the first edition of this text is the changing conception of the validity of educational tests and measures (e.g., rubrics, clinical evaluation tools). In this chapter, we adopt the definition of validity provided in the most recent edition of the *Standards for Educational and Psychological Testing* (AERA, APA, & NCME, 2014), which notes that "validity refers to the degree to which evidence and theory support the interpretation of test scores for proposed uses of tests" (p. 11). This conception of validity represents a shift away from the more traditional, research-oriented definition (i.e., validity is the extent to which a scale/test measures what it claims to measure) to a contextually focused definition, championed most successfully by Messick (1995). Messick emphasized the nature of validity as a unitary construct that, while inclusive of the traditional types of validity evidence (i.e., content, construct, and criterion), should be more intently focused on *validity as a process* or ongoing *argument* that must be continuously evaluated and supported.

In a recent qualitative exploration of the different (and sometimes divergent) *validity narratives* in the scholarly literature, St-Onge, Young, Eva, and Hodges (2017) described the now-disfavored traditional view of validity and reliability as one where validity and reliability are relatively stable characteristics of a measure or exam, which suggests validity and reliability can be "established." This view, however widely held (evidenced by statements such as "the tool was valid and reliable..."), is inconsistent with the very nature of the research evidence that supports claims of validity and reliability. Specifically, the research evidence used to support measurement validity and reliability claims is subject to the same threats, biases, and limitations as every other type of research—but is somehow treated more preferentially, and perhaps uncritically. The central limitation is that all study findings and conclusions are based on data from a specific sample used in a study: findings related to the tool's construct validity, internal consistency reliability, or any dimension of measure performance are thusly highly sample specific and context dependent.

The recognition of this fundamental limitation on what can be inferred from any measure of human subjects led to development of what St-Onge et al. call the *process-focused* validity narrative championed by Messick and, in large part, adopted in the most recent standards (AERA, APA, & NCME, 2014). This validity narrative focuses more strongly on the process of continuously developing and evaluating the evidence to support the intended uses of an educational test or measure. For example, a standardized test developed to predict student success in college should not be used for other purposes, such as to identify students in need of subject-specific remediation, without sufficient theoretical and empirical evidence to support that additional use of the test.

Likewise, to make defensible, trustworthy inferences from students' test scores, normative data from demographically similar students must be available—an inherently difficult challenge for all but the largest of large-scale assessment programs to achieve. For readers interested in a more detailed review of the historical development of validity theory over the past seven decades, both Kane (2006) and Moss, Girard, and Haniford (2006) provide detailed, seminal accounts.

While conceptions of educational test and measurement validity have noticeably evolved over the last decade, conceptions of test *reliability* have remained relatively stable, with some caveats. Reliability is most closely aligned with the terms *accuracy*, *precision*, and *consistency*—all terms that indicate how predictable, constant, and reproducible the results of measurements are, either internally (e.g., internal consistent reliability) or from one measurement to the next (e.g., test-retest reliability; Lane et al., 2016; McDonald, 2014). Validity and reliability are related concepts, and the dictum learned in any course on research methods or tests and measurements still stands (even with evolutions in validity theory): reliability is a necessary, but not sufficient, condition for validity. That is, a test must demonstrate strong reliability for a validity argument to be made. However, tests can show evidence of reliability (i.e., consistency), but not validity, in that a test can consistently and precisely measure its construct, but if the construct is misrecognized or misinterpreted by the educator or researcher using the test, validity arguments made from it can be incorrect. For example, if an educator uses an anxiety measure designed to measure trait anxiety (i.e., anxiety that is dispositional rather than situational in nature) before and after a classroom test-anxiety reduction intervention, interpretations of the anxiety scores may be incorrect because the instrument measures something other than what the educator intended to measure. In this hypothetical situation, the instrument could show strong internal consistency reliability, and even strong test-retest reliability, but the interpretations—which hinge on the instrument's validity for the intended use—are likely to be erroneous given that the construct of interest, situational test anxiety, was not measured by the trait anxiety tool.

A full discussion of how the reliability of a test or measure is evaluated is beyond the scope of this chapter; readers are referred to Oermann and Gaberson (2014) or Thorndike and Thorndike-Christ (2011) for more complete discussion. Here, in support of evidence-based assessment and evaluation decision-making, several important considerations relevant to evaluating a test or measure's reliability claims are provided. First, while the most commonly reported index of instrument reliability is its internal consistency reliability, usually estimated using a Cronbach's alpha (also called *coefficient alpha*), this measure of reliability is not appropriate for some types of measures. And, because alpha is highly influenced by sample size and scale length, the internal consistency of measures can either be over- or underestimated depending on whether sample sizes are large or small (Spurlock, 2016).

On the issue of appropriate application of Cronbach's alpha, only in cases where there is a theoretical basis for instrument responses to be internally consistent is it appropriate to use alpha as a measure of internal consistency. For example, it would be appropriate to evaluate alpha for a 10-item instrument measuring students' leadership self-efficacy because the construct of interest is narrow enough and the response scale (likely a Likert or Likert-type scale) is appropriate to support its use. For educators interested in the reliability of multiple-choice exams, which can cover many different areas of content knowledge and for which the responses are not provided on a continuous response scale, Cronbach's alpha is not an appropriate choice. Educators might consider split-half or parallel forms methods to evaluate test reliability in these cases (Thorndike & Thorndike-Christ, 2011).

On the issue of the sensitivity of alpha to sample size, an admonition similar to the one presented earlier about the fallibility of validity and reliability study findings is in order. That is, even in contexts where Cronbach's alpha is an appropriate method to evaluate the reliability of a test or measure, if sample sizes are too small (as is often the case when measures are taken in classrooms of 15 to 25 students), reliability estimates will be imprecise; the same considerations of statistical power apply to calculations of Cronbach's alpha just as with any other statistical test (Tavakol & Dennick, 2011). Similarly, Cronbach's alpha favors longer scales over shorter ones, which generally results in higher alpha estimates for longer scales, even when administered to small groups of individuals.

With these considerations in mind, nurse educators can make more accurate decisions about test or scale reliability than if relying only on simplistic but arbitrarily established cut-offs, such as Cronbach's alpha = .70, to assess the reliability evidence for a given test or assessment. Recognizing the limitations of Cronbach's alpha and other statistical estimates of scale reliability is a fundamental skill for nurse educators, made exceptionally accessible for educators by the widespread availability of item analysis software and the reference texts mentioned earlier in the chapter. In sum, a robust understanding of the modern, ethically and empirically informed conceptions of measurement validity and reliability enables nurse educators to use tests and other measures in defensible, evidence-based ways, expressed clearly in the task statements of *Competency III* from the *Scope of Practice for Academic Nurse Educators* (NLN, 2012c).

Assessment and Evaluation of Learning in the Cognitive Domain

The cognitive learning domain includes both content knowledge and thinking skills, as well as the integration between these two inseparable dimensions of cognition. Nurse educators evaluate learning in the cognitive domain primarily through the use of both teacher-developed and commercially available tests of content knowledge. Most of the attention in the nursing education literature during the reviewed period (2005 to 2017) has focused on test-related topics, while less attention has been paid to assessment and evaluation of critical thinking, clinical reasoning, and decision-making skills.

In a significant contribution to the nursing education literature, Oermann, Saewert, Charasika, and Yarbrough (2009) reported results from a survey of the assessment and evaluation practices of 1,573 prelicensure nurse faculty from across the United States. Across all types of prelicensure RN programs, written papers, group projects, case studies, care plans, and exams (both teacher developed and standardized) were the most frequently reported methods to assess learning in the cognitive domain. Oermann, Saewert, et al. reported that though nonexam methods were among the most commonly used assessment and evaluation methods, 57 percent of faculty respondents reported that exams counted the most toward course grades. Faculty respondents also reported that NCLEX-RN pass rates were the primary driving factor in the choice of assessment and evaluation strategies. Given the immense importance and focus by nursing education programs on the nursing licensure examination pass rates, the correspondingly strong focus on tests and examinations in prelicensure programs is not unexpected.

Because such important, often high-stakes decisions are made based on students' test scores, nurse educators must ensure the tests they use have been developed using well-accepted, best-practice approaches. Comprehensive, evidence-based guidance on local development of tests and exams (sometimes called teacher-developed tests) can be found in reference texts such as McDonald (2014) and Oermann and Gaberson (2014), among other sources previously identified. In addition, the test item writing principles provided by Haladyna, Downing, and Rodriguez (2002), which include a summary of the previous two decades' worth of empirical evidence supporting each of the 31 test item writing principles, remain relevant and instructive despite having been published in 2002. An example item writing principle that may be of interest to nurse educators is that with multiple-choice test items, three-answer options (instead of four) provide greater efficiency for the test taker without losing any power to discriminate between students who know and those who do not know the content being tested (Haladyna et al., 2002).

Nursing-education-focused, data-based literature directly related to test item development, administration, or evaluation of teacher-developed tests during the reviewed period is quite limited. Selected papers, presented chronologically, include first a study by Sandahl (2010) of collaborative testing among a sample of 110 prelicensure nursing students. Sandahl found that students testing in collaborative settings generally scored 2 to 4 points higher than students taking nursing content exams individually. Because the study used a nonexperimental crossover design, where all subjects participated in group testing for some of the tests in the course and no students participated in group testing for final exams, finding that no statistically or practically significant differences were observed in final course grades makes evaluation of any learning benefit difficult to assess. In studying the issue of test anxiety and the impact it has on exam performance, Brodersen (2017), in a recent integrative review of the literature, synthesized findings from 33 studies of test-anxiety reduction interventions among nursing students from 1973 to 2014. Brodersen found limited but high-quality evidence for aromatherapy, music therapy, and other cognitive interventions; nonexperimental studies have supported other less common strategies, such as collaborative testing, use of crib sheets, and humor.

High-Stakes Testing in Classroom Settings

A more fruitful area of inquiry and publication in nursing education research from 2005 to 2017 has been around the issue of high-stakes testing in nursing education, including the use of commercially available comprehensive standardized nursing exit tests to make progression or graduation decisions. Following research published in late 2004 (Spurlock & Hanks, 2004), Spurlock (2006) identified important considerations for nurse educators who use commercially available standardized tests, including the importance of situating high-stakes decision-making within recognized ethical and technical guidelines, such as those provided (in their most current form) by the AERA, APA, and NCME (2014), and the need to focus on the issue of test-use validity, a term used in the mid-2000s to refer to validity evidence supporting the intended uses of tests and measures.

Continuing the same line of inquiry, which established the importance of evaluating how well high-stakes tests predict both licensure exam success and failure, Spurlock and

Hunt (2008) examined the predictive accuracy of a standardized exit exam on the NCLEX-RN outcomes of a sample of 179 baccalaureate nursing students. The researchers found that while high scores on the exit exam were associated with positive (passing) outcomes on the NCLEX-RN, low exit exam scores did not reliably predict student failure. That is, even students scoring in the lowest scoring categories assigned by the exit exam passed the NCLEX-RN exam, on average, more than 70 percent of the time. Spurlock and Hunt also found that the correlations between exit exam scores and the NCLEX-RN outcomes diminished with each repeat administration of the exit exam, indicating that repeat exit exam scores were less predictive than the scores from the first administration of the exit exam.

Harding (2010), in a review of the literature on the predictability of exit exams, reached the same conclusion as Spurlock and Hanks (2004) and Spurlock and Hunt (2008), finding that while high exit exam scores indicate a strong probability of passing the NCLEX-RN, the licensure exam outcomes for low scorers cannot be reliably predicted by exit exam scores alone. Brodersen and Mills (2014), using regression and diagnostic accuracy procedures and methods similar to those of Spurlock and Hunt (2008), replicated the findings of Spurlock and Hunt among a sample of 317 prelicensure baccalaureate nursing students. Brodersen and Mills reported correlations of $r = .34$ to .36 between NCLEX-RN outcomes and exit exam scores, and correspondingly low classification accuracy (18.2 percent correct prediction rate) for students with low exit exam scores who were predicted to fail the NCLEX-RN. These findings support the need for continuing vigilance on the part of nurse educators involved with evaluating commercial testing products for use in nursing education programs to ensure that, in alignment with *Competency III* from the *Scope of Practice for Academic Nurse Educators* (NLN, 2012c), educators use these tests in ways that are supported by a strong evidence base.

The rise in the use of commercially available standardized nursing-content exams during the 2000s and findings from research (discussed earlier) that call into question the validity of such exams for high-stakes decision-making (Spurlock, 2013) led to a national dialogue among nursing education leaders and professional organizations. One outcome of those discussions was the development of nursing-education-specific fair testing guidelines by the NLN (NLN 2012a, 2012b). These guidelines make it clear that substantial evidence should support the intended uses of tests, especially when the stakes are high for students, and that important educational decisions—such as whether a student will graduate or not—should not be made on the basis of a single test score, especially when so many other indicators of student achievement and capability are readily accessible to nurse educators. The NLN Fair Testing Guidelines are consistent with the recently updated *Standards for Educational and Psychological Testing* (AERA, APA, & NCME, 2014), providing further support for the wide adoption of the NLN Fair Testing Guidelines by nurse educators.

Critical Thinking, Clinical Reasoning, and Clinical Judgment

The last area of cognitive domain assessment and evaluation covered in this section deals with thinking and reasoning skills, with the terms *critical thinking* and *clinical reasoning* being the most commonly used technical terms in the nursing education literature. The nursing education literature from 2005 to 2017 reveals that little progress has been made in both the conceptualization and measurement of critical thinking in nursing education, a problem that has persisted for decades despite the long-time inclusion of critical thinking as an essential student learning outcome in nursing education programs in the United States (Riddel, 2007; Walsh & Seldomridge, 2006).

Several literature reviews and synthesis papers highlight the challenges of measuring and evaluating critical thinking, including the lack of agreement on a conceptual definition of critical thinking, the poor validity and reliability evidence for critical thinking tools, and inadequate statistical and psychometric reporting in studies of critical thinking among nursing students (Carter, Creedy, & Sidebotham, 2015; Nair & Stamler, 2013; Romeo, 2010). The findings from nursing education are echoed in papers exploring the assessment and evaluation of critical thinking in higher education more generally (see, e.g., Liu, Frankel, & Roohr, 2014). To illustrate some of these challenges, Searing and Kooken (2016), in a study of 96 prelicensure nursing students, found low, nonsignificant correlations between students' scores on one widely used tool, the California Critical Thinking Disposition Inventory (CCTDI), and multiple other student learning outcome variables including science course grades, program completion, standardized exit exam scores, and NCLEX-RN success. Similarly, Shirrell (2008) found that though grade point average was a weak but statistically significant predictor, students' scores on the Collegiate Assessment of Academic Proficiency, a critical thinking test, did not predict NCLEX-RN success among a sample of 173 prelicensure nursing students enrolled in an associate degree program. Findings from these few example studies echo those of a multitude of other studies conducted over the previous three decades, creating significant doubt about the utility of additional studies focused on critical thinking, especially given the continuing challenges with conceptualization and measurement of the concept.

Perhaps reflecting an evolution of thinking among some nursing education researchers in response to the decades-long inquiry into critical thinking in nursing, a renewed focus on clinical judgment and reasoning has come into focus over the last 10 to 15 years. This focus is exemplified by models of clinical reasoning and judgment proposed principally by Pesut and Herman (1999) and Tanner (2006). Bartlett et al. (2008) described the usefulness of the Outcome-Present State-Test (OPT) Model of clinical reasoning developed from the original work by Pesut and Herman (1999). The OPT model was conceptualized to include both a visual/mental framework for developing clinical reasoning skills and pedagogical approaches to helping students develop those skills. In the OPT model, the nursing student identifies cues relevant to the patient's condition, uses reflection to frame the cues, and then develops strategies to help move the patient toward the desired outcome state. Bartlett et al. described using the OPT model via vignette-based case studies where students were encouraged to reason through the steps to take patients from their present clinical state to the desired health outcome state. The OPT model provided scripting along the way to help students identify important clinical issues and consider, more holistically, the kinds of information essential to their own clinical decision-making. While evaluation and adoption of the OPT model are somewhat limited at present, it provides a potential avenue for further research and testing that extends beyond what seems possible by continuing pursuits of ill-defined critical thinking outcomes.

Tanner (2006) presented a research-based model of clinical reasoning from a highly social-cognitive perspective, using terms easily understood by nurse educators and students alike. Tanner outlined five assumptions about the nature of nurses' clinical reasoning and judgments: (1) clinical judgments are impacted more by the nurse's prior experience than by the subjective data available to the nurse; (2) clinical judgments are best when they include knowledge of the patient and the patient's health patterns, as well as engagement with the patient's concerns; (3) the care setting—its context and culture—impact clinical judgments and decision-making; (4) nurses do not use one reasoning pattern alone to make clinical judgments but use multiple patterns, sometimes in combination; and (5) reflection is critical for the development of skills in clinical judgment but is often not triggered until deficits in clinical judgment occur.

A recent systematic review (Cappelletti, Engel, & Prentice, 2014) of the literature found continuing support for the tenants of Tanner's (2006) clinical judgment model, with consideration for adding an additional contextual factor (addressing the impact of educational experiences) beyond what was specified in the original model. Following publication of the Tanner model in 2006, Lasater (2007) developed the Lasater Clinical Judgment Rubric (LCJR) (described more fully later) as a practical tool for educators and students to use in evaluating the extent to which students engaged in model-based behaviors (e.g., noticing, interpreting) during simulation learning experiences. This work was followed by additional development and testing in the context of concept-based learning activities (Lasater & Nielsen, 2009), and studies comparing the correspondence between faculty and student evaluations of clinical judgment using the LCJR, which were found to be strong (Strickland, Cheshire, & March, 2017). Kavanagh and Szweda (2017) described plans to implement Tanner's (2006) clinical judgment model and use the LCJR with high-fidelity simulations at the Cleveland Clinic to evaluate and improve the clinical reasoning skills of new graduate RNs, in conjunction with continuing use of a commercially available, Internet-based clinical reasoning skills evaluation system. In sum, the Tanner (2006) model continues to prompt a fruitful line of inquiry and scholarship that impacts nursing education and practice more than a decade after its initial publication. It also illustrates how, consistent with *Competency III* from the *Scope of Practice for Academic Nurse Educators* (NLN, 2012c), educators might improve their practices of developing and using tools to evaluate clinical practice by designing these tools based on relevant theoretical and empirical models.

Assessment and Evaluation of Learning in the Psychomotor Domain

The goal of nursing education is to graduate safe and competent practitioners who are well positioned to care for people in an ever-changing health care environment. Evaluating clinical competence is multifaceted and involves the assessment of psychomotor skills, the application of theoretical knowledge, clinical judgment, and the ability to respond to changing situations (Walsh & Seldomridge, 2005). Rigorous assessment and evaluation of clinical performance by nurse educators are essential in preparing nursing students to enter into the nursing workforce in any setting. Tools with strong validity and reliability evidence help nurse educators ensure that the student is competent and safe to enter practice (Oermann, Yarbrough, Saewert, Ard, & Charasika, 2009) and facilitate communication between faculty and students (Shipman, Roa, Hooten, & Wang, 2012). While many nurses will practice in the acute care setting, nurses enter the workforce in a diverse range of settings. All too often, evaluation in the clinical and simulation setting focuses only on the psychomotor domain and lacks attention to critical thinking, decision-making, problem solving, teamwork, communication, and collaboration. Nurse educators need to develop competence in evaluating student learning outcomes related to these essential aspects of professional nursing care. Findings from several studies reporting to measure higher order clinical performance are highlighted next. Findings from these studies are consistent with other findings and reports in the literature and have demonstrated growing acceptance among nurse educators.

Simulation-Based High-Stakes Testing

Simulation is frequently used as an educational strategy in nursing education. However, for simulation to be effective, it is critical that best practice guidelines be observed (Cant & Cooper, 2010), especially when summative assessment and high-stakes evaluation are being used. As a teaching strategy, simulation is typically depicted as presenting a safe learning environment where students can practice and make mistakes; high-stakes testing in simulation can remove the feeling of safety, making it imperative to use evidence-based approaches and collaboration for scenario development for student evaluation (Willhaus, Burleson, Palaganas, & Jeffries, 2014). High-stakes evaluation is defined as "an evaluation process associated with a simulation activity that has a major academic, education, or employment consequence (such as a grading decision, including pass or fail implications; a decision regarding competency, merit pay, promotion, or certification). High stakes refers to the outcome or consequences of the process" (Meakim et al., 2013, p. S7).

The use of simulation for high-stakes evaluation continues to evolve, and with well-written, rigorously evaluated scenarios, higher order thinking and clinical judgment can be assessed (Boulet, Murray, Kras, & Woodhouse, 2008; Rutherford-Hemming, Kardong-Edgren, Gore, Ravert, & Rizzolo, 2014). In spring 2014, in a survey of 605 undergraduate and hospital educators, 42 percent reported using high-fidelity simulations, and 28 percent reported using objective structured clinical examinations (OSCEs) for high-stakes assessment (Rutherford-Hemming et al., 2014). Through additional discussion, questions were raised about the quality control of the practices used during the high-stakes testing.

Experts in simulation have weighed in on the use of high-stakes testing. Ravert (in Rutherford-Hemming et al., 2014) reported that though the use of simulation for summative assessment is increasing, in many nursing education programs, simulation is still used primarily as a formative methodology. Ravert raised some concerns about the defensibility of high-stakes testing and cautioned that if high-stakes testing is to be used, scenarios should be validated and the simulation-based high-stakes testing should be part of a larger assessment plan. Rizzolo (in Rutherford-Hemming et al., 2014) noted that the difficulty in implementing fair testing practices cannot be overlooked; although high-stakes testing in simulation may be difficult to implement, it may lead to more fair and equitable evaluation processes. Gore (in Rutherford-Hemming et al., 2014) emphasized the need for validated scenarios, instruments with strong validity and reliability evidence for use in evaluating student performance, and the proper "dose" of simulation to realize the best outcome. Kardong-Edgren, Oermann, Rizzolo, and Odom-Maryon (2017) emphasized the importance of rater training and establishing interrater reliability for evaluators who are involved in high-stakes testing.

Clinical and Simulation-Based Rubrics

A rubric is a scoring instrument or tool used to assess or evaluate a student's ability to meet or exceed certain criteria or objectives; although much of the literature on rubrics focuses on clinical or simulation settings, nurse educators can employ well-developed and tested rubrics in other settings such as the classroom or on discussion boards in the online learning environment. When developed effectively, rubrics can be an effective method of assessment and evaluation; however, poorly constructed rubrics can provide unreliable and biased feedback, especially in the clinical setting (Shipman et al., 2012). In developing rubrics for scoring in the clinical or simulated environment, nurse educators must adhere to the principles of well-constructed rubrics (Stevens, Levi, & Walvoord, 2012) with a rating scale to determine exactly how well the student met the criteria or objectives. These well-developed and tested rubrics can be used by nurse educators to assess student performance and provide meaningful and constructive feedback when applied consistently, facilitating student learning and growth (Lasater, 2011; Shipman et al., 2012; Stevens et al., 2012).

Oermann, Yarbrough, et al. (2009) found that 37 percent of prelicensure programs use rubrics as a clinical evaluation method; however, they noted that nurse educators should exercise caution when using rubrics that are not research tested, especially if students are receiving a grade. The Lasater Clinical Judgment Rubric (LCJR) (2007) provides an example of an assessment rubric founded on Tanner's (2006) clinical judgment model. It uses the four elements (with 11 dimensions) of critical thinking that Tanner defined as essential: noticing, interpreting, responding, and reflecting. While the LCJR has been used in multiple settings and studies (Adamson, 2011; Ashcraft et al., 2013; Gubrud-Howe, 2008; Jensen, 2013; Manetti, 2015; Mariani, Cantrell, Meakim, Prieto, & Dreifuerst, 2013), a significant amount of its use has been in simulated learning environments, where it has been demonstrated to be an effective, evidence-based clinical judgment rubric that can be used to help prelicensure students think like a nurse (Lasater, 2011). The LCJR was created using sound principles of rubric development (Shipman at al., 2012; Stevens et al., 2012) and provides educators with a well-tested assessment tool.

Nurse educators can incorporate principles from *Competency III* from the *Scope of Practice for Academic Nurse Educators* (NLN, 2012c), improving educators' practices in developing and using tools to evaluate clinical practice, as they develop and use rubrics to assess and evaluate students in a variety of settings. Rubrics provide a level playing field for all students, as well as a means of communication between students and faculty, where all parties are using common language (Lasater, 2007).

Clinical Assessment Tools

Oermann, Yarbrough, et al. (2009) reported on a survey conducted by the NLN Evaluation of Learning Advisory Council to better understand how educators grade and evaluate clinical practice of nursing students. From the large sample size of 1,573 nurse educators from across many types of prelicensure RN programs, 98 percent reported using some type of clinical evaluation tool in the clinical setting; 83 percent reported using a pass/fail grading scale; and 70 percent reported using the same basic rating scale for all courses, with some variations from course to course. Oermann, Yarbrough, et al. listed several limitations with the study, such as limited study sample demographics, the inability to calculate a response rate, and a lack of reliability with the survey tool. In conclusion, they noted that many inconsistencies exist in clinical grading among faculty.

In an example of this concern, Walsh and Seldomridge (2005) studied the relationship between paired clinical and theory grades and found evidence of clinical grade inflation. Walsh and Seldomridge described some of the possible reasons as broad clinical performance expectations, differences in evaluation of theory and clinical expectations, the "Rule of C" (where C is almost seen as a failing grade), the inability for faculty to see everything in the clinical setting, role effort as part of the grade, the recency of the performance, and lack of thorough anecdotal records. These findings should highlight for nurse educators the many considerations necessary to rigorously assess and evaluate clinical learning, even when using rubrics or other structured approaches.

In an innovative recent example from outside the United States, Skúladottir and Svavarsdottir (2016) developed and reported initial validity evidence for the Clinical Assessment Tool for Nursing Education (CAT-NE) to guide students' clinical education and to evaluate their clinical performance. The rubric, which includes a list of expected clinical behaviors, as well as student self-assessment and the clinical faculty's evaluation, was designed to clarify learning objectives, enhance the focus of the assessment process, and make the evaluation process more objective. In developing the CAT-NE, Skúladottir and Svavarsdottir gathered validity evidence by using content experts, expert teachers, clinical faculty, and students. They also provided a training session for raters prior to its use. Since this tool was only used in one setting, it needs further testing. However, the CAT-NE illustrates the possibility of developing more objective, evidence-based instruments, critical for evaluating clinical learning and performance.

Concept Mapping in Clinical and Simulated Settings

Critical thinking, clinical judgment, problem solving, and decision-making are crucial skills that prelicensure nursing students must develop to be safe and competent practitioners. Concept maps are diagrammatic representations of the student's thought processes that include links and relationships among and between concepts. The process of concept mapping may stimulate critical thinking by helping to make meaning of concepts using deductive or inductive thinking skills (Gul & Boman, 2006). It can be valuable in promoting the complex thought processes (Stewart, 2011) that are often necessary in the clinical setting.

Daley, Morgan, and Black's (2016) historical literature review found that concept maps have been used in nursing education for approximately 25 years to help students gain meaningful learning by ordering, distinguishing, differentiating, and analyzing concepts in ways in which they can be synthesized to represent an integrated whole. There has been a large body of work to inform the use of concept maps, and an increasing body of evidence-based literature supports concept maps in promoting critical thinking and clinical judgment. However, gaps exist in understanding the theoretical connectedness of the concept map to learning, the development of scoring models and formulas to evaluate concept maps, and the impact of concept mapping on learning.

Gerdeman, Lux, and Jacko's (2013) qualitative study of eight undergraduate nursing students evaluated concept mapping exercises in developing critical thinking skills, understanding the clinical situation, and developing clinical judgment skills. Although the sample size was small, students reported that the concept mapping activity and rubric contributed to helping them make better clinical decisions. They also felt it increased their clinical judgment skills. Continuing this line of inquiry, Yeo (2014) conducted a literature review on concept maps and critical thinking, identifying eight factors affecting the successful implementation of concept mapping to improve critical thinking. These eight factors were identified as learners' ability, facilitators, types of concept maps, context, clear instruction, focus on learning, explanations, and appropriateness of timing.

Chen, Liang, Li, and Liao (2011) conducted a quasi-experimental study to explore the differences in critical thinking ability in prelicensure undergraduate nursing students who used concept maps as a method of learning in comparison to students who learned from lecture. Although this study was not conducted in the clinical setting, the findings included evidence of a statistically significant improvement in critical thinking scores for the group that used concept maps.

These four studies (Chen et al., 2011; Daley et al., 2016; Gerdeman et al., 2013; Yeo, 2014) clearly provide support for the use of concept maps as a teaching/learning strategy in nursing education, especially in developing critical thinking. However, they also identify the need for nurse educators to generate more evidence for concept maps to further their use in the assessment and evaluation of nursing students.

Assessment and Evaluation of Learning in the Affective Domain

Of the three learning domains (cognitive, psychomotor, and affective) used to organize this chapter, assessment and evaluation of learning in the affective domain have received the least attention in the nursing education literature since the first edition of this text. Where the term *affective* relates generally to one's feelings and emotions, the assessment of learning in the affective domain involves examining students' skill development and capability in areas including professional values, beliefs, and attitudes. The importance of addressing learning in the affective domain was highlighted by Valiga (2014, p. 247), who noted, "When we devote extensive—and sometimes all—class time to covering content and focusing curriculum discussions more on *what they need to know* than on *who they need to become*, we are undermining the opportunity to prepare our students to be the leaders, scholars, perpetual learners, and active members of the profession our future and the public need them to be."

The review of the nursing education literature from 2005 to 2017 illustrates that while constructs clearly situated within the affective domain are not infrequently studied by nursing education researchers, the extent to which nurse educators regularly assess and evaluate these constructs among their students, for primarily educational purposes, remains disappointingly low, a point noted by Taylor (2014). In a study of 69 accelerated BSN students, Ward (2015) examined the effect of a brief simulation-based educational intervention on students' attitudes toward mental health patients' experiences of hearing voices. Data were generated before and after the administration of the Medical

Condition Regards Scale (MCRS), a self-report attitudes and beliefs instrument, and through analysis of students' narrative comments provided in their evaluation of the simulation experience. Overall results showed improvement in MCRS scores on several items, and the students' narrative comments reflected satisfaction and increased sensitivity to patients with serious mental illness.

Amerson (2012) investigated the impact of an intercultural, international service-learning trip on students' ($n = 22$) transcultural self-efficacy. Amerson detailed the overall positive impact of the service-learning experience on students' awareness, recognition, and understanding of the impact of culture on health, and of students' comfort with providing culturally sensitive care. Likewise, Wellmon, Lefebvre, and Ferry (2017) examined the effect of a brief, interprofessional mock code simulation involving both nursing ($n = 35$) and physical therapy students ($n = 42$) on students' attitudes toward interprofessional learning and teamwork, among other variables. Wellmon et al. reported positive improvements in students' attitudes and perceptions, for both nursing and physical therapy students, in the postintervention period. The findings of these studies provide initial evidence of the effects of relatively brief educational interventions, but studies taking a more longitudinal approach—likely necessary for sustaining a durable impact on attitudes and beliefs—are needed.

In what is perhaps the first published description of a formal academic course designed specifically to address the affective domain, Day et al. (2017) described the development and implementation of a course delivered to 68 prelicensure nursing students at four schools of nursing in the United States. The course was organized around activities designed to promote self-reflection and the development of beliefs and values central to the profession of nursing. Faculty members coordinating the course and students who participated in the course evaluated the experience in a positive manner, with students strongly confirming that the course offered them opportunities not provided elsewhere in the curriculum. This innovative approach, where an entire, structured course, designed to target development in the affective domain, is worthy of further study and evaluation, especially where measures and further qualitative exploration of nursing-specific values and attitude development can be undertaken.

While leaders in both nursing education (Valiga, 2014) and practice (Jones-Schenk, 2016) have indicated the importance of a renewed focus on affective learning, several issues could explain the relatively infrequent assessment and evaluation of affective learning by nurse educators. These include the lack of agreement on a common set of affective learning outcomes for nursing education programs, the lack of available measures to easily and efficiently measure affective constructs, and, even if those measures exist, hesitation within nursing education programs to add more measures to an already lengthy list of required tests, surveys, and evaluations. Despite these challenges, researchers have demonstrated that nurse educators can impact affective learning outcomes and that affective learning can be evaluated, as highlighted in the papers reviewed previously.

IDENTIFIED GAPS IN THE LITERATURE

Like the nursing education research literature more generally, the literature supporting the development of faculty competencies associated with assessment and evaluation practices in nursing education has remained quite limited during the 2005–2017 period.

The majority of nursing education research continues to be statistically underpowered, conducted within a single site, and is hampered by the lack of available measures with sufficient validity and reliability evidence. Studies also suffer from other common problems related to the quality of statistical reporting: missing (but essential) details such as basic subject demographic information necessary for evaluating generalizability and external validity, and the continuing reliance on highly subjective measures (such as self-report), even when more objective methods of measurement are available. Nursing education researchers must focus on addressing these general issues moving forward if the field is to develop a robust evidence base for nurse educator practice.

Within the cognitive domain of learning, little research is available to guide commonly made assessment and evaluation decisions. Little or no nursing-education-specific empirical evidence exists to support the frequency of administering knowledge tests, ideal test length, mode of test administration (e.g., test versus computerized administration), and item construction. Nurse educators continue to rely on tradition, conventions, and evidence extrapolated from other fields to guide their decision-making. Too many nursing education research studies continue to examine the relationship between primarily cognitive predictors, such as academic course grades and standardized test scores, and NCLEX-RN outcomes, when decades of studies on this topic have failed to find useful signals amid the substantial noise produced, in large part, by within- and between-program variability. Missing from the literature are well-developed lines of inquiry that explore how metacognitive, noncognitive, social, socioeconomic, and other variables of interest contribute to nursing student success on the NCLEX—and beyond. Also notably missing from the literature are high-quality studies that inform assessment of student writing skills and abilities, at both the undergraduate and graduate levels.

Within the psychomotor domain of learning, questions remain about the most effective methods of evaluating clinical skill acquisition and maintenance. Nurse educators lack basic normative data on the amounts and types of instruction, practice, and feedback required for students to acquire new psychomotor skills of varying complexity. Likewise, the literature does not provide adequate support about the ideal intervals and methods for assessing continuing clinical skill maintenance among students (and practicing nurses), and many studies still continue to focus on self-confidence and satisfaction. Are the clinical skills that prelicensure students acquire and demonstrate early in their programs sufficiently maintained during the course of the program, to promote both patient safety and new-graduate practice readiness? Likewise, the same questions and concerns exist for graduate students, especially in programs preparing students for advanced practice roles. How can nurse educators most efficiently and effectively evaluate skill acquisition and maintenance?

As was noted previously, the affective domain presents perhaps the most opportunity for future research and knowledge development. Though nursing education researchers frequently study variables falling within the affective domain (e.g., self-efficacy, satisfaction, beliefs), evidence to support the selection of and methods of measurement of affective variables in educational settings is markedly lacking. Studies that use time-intensive methods to examine affective variables, such as extensive interview procedures or self-report survey measures with little demonstrated ecological validity, provide little help to nurse educators interested primarily in student- and program-level student learning outcomes. New methods, measures, and conceptual frameworks—preferably focusing on the observable behaviors produced by the presence of desirable professional nursing values, beliefs, and attitudes—are sorely needed.

In reviewing the research priorities for assessment and evaluation strategies outlined in the first edition of this text, our assessment of the extent to which the literature has substantially helped answer the questions is mixed. In many ways, such as with high-stakes testing and the expanded use of simulation-based evaluation, aspects of what would constitute "best practices" are beginning to emerge. But the evidence base continues to lack the depth necessary to qualify as a strong evidentiary foundation. Further, as readers may detect in reading this chapter, the attention paid in the literature to assessment and evaluation in graduate nursing education is disproportionately low, especially given the rapid growth in these programs over the past two decades. In terms of evaluating competence, another priority research question identified in the first edition of this text, this subject too has produced mixed results. Nursing education still has no well-accepted definition of competence and, correspondingly, no well-accepted method to evaluate it. Educators in other health professions fields, most notably in medicine, have begun their extraction from the "competency quagmire" by developing a new paradigm focused on *entrustable professional activities* (Carraccio et al., 2017), which asks educators not to deem a student *competent*, but to answer the question "Can the student be trusted to perform a given professional activity, and at what level of supervision?" Nursing could be well served by exploring this newly developed framework, perhaps in support of a needed paradigm shift in nursing.

Other questions asked in the previous edition of this text dealt with the utility and best practices around the use of concept mapping to promote critical thinking, and portfolios and journaling to evaluate student learning. These formative assessment strategies were perhaps of more interest to both educators and those contributing to the nursing education literature during the time period covered in the first edition of this text than they are today. While concept mapping and journaling are still in wide use, portfolios seem to have evolved more into vehicles to present a corpus of work than as a product with great formative assessment value. Lastly, apart from one notable large-scale study examining prelicensure student learning outcomes when up to 50 percent of clinical time was replaced by simulation experiences (National Council of State Boards of Nursing, 2014), we still know little about the most effective structures (frequency, required number of hours, etc.) to promote optimal student learning outcomes among prelicensure clinical nursing students—and we know even less about these same questions among graduate students enrolled in APRN preparation programs.

PRIORITIES FOR FUTURE RESEARCH

Based on the review of the literature presented here and emergent trends in nursing education, the following list of topical and methodological priorities for assessment and evaluation-related nursing education research have been identified:

> ▸ High-stakes testing and assessment remains a salient issue for nurse educators at all levels of nursing education. What is the role of contextual factors such as student characteristics, faculty experience with high-stakes assessment, and the rapidly changing nature of the health care system in establishing and continuously evaluating the validity and reliability claims for these types of assessments?

➤ Given the limited literature in this area of simulation, what role should standardized patients play across all levels of nursing education? Additionally, as emerging technologies such as headset-based virtual reality become more widely available, to what extent are these technologies effective and comparable to existing forms of simulation-based learning?

➤ What are the optimal methods and procedures for assessment and evaluation relevant to graduate nursing education, and to APRN education in particular?

➤ How do the advancements made in clinical *implementation science* intersect with nursing education in terms of both curriculum and how nurse educators can better discover, understand, and implement research and other forms of evidence into their practice as educators?

➤ How can nurse educators and nursing education researchers best collaborate toward ensuring that the methods, procedures, and measures used in assessment- and evaluation-related research can be replicated or applied beyond the sites used in individual studies?

➤ What are the barriers and facilitators nurse educators face in using assessment and evaluation methods that are (1) more objective, rather than subjective, in nature and (2) most directly measure the variable of interest (i.e., measuring the variable of direct interest, like *actual skill performance*, is preferred to measuring a surrogate variable, such as *confidence in skill performance*)?

References

Adamson, K. A. (2011). *Assessing the reliability of simulation evaluation instruments used in nursing education: A test of concept study* (Doctoral dissertation). Retrieved from Pro-Quest Dissertations and Theses database. (UMI No. 3460357)

American Educational Research Association, American Psychological Association, & National Council on Measurement in Education. (2014). *Standards for educational and psychological testing* (3rd ed.). Washington, DC: American Educational Research Association.

Amerson, R. (2012). The influence of international service-learning on transcultural self-efficacy in baccalaureate nursing graduates and their subsequent practice. *International Journal of Teaching and Learning in Higher Education, 24*(1), 6–15.

Ashcraft, A. S., Opton, L., Bridges, R. A., Caballero, S., Veesart, A., & Weaver, C. (2013). Simulation evaluation using a modified Lasater Clinical Judgment Rubric. *Nursing Education Perspectives, 34*, 122–126.

Bartlett, R., Bland, A., Rossen, E., Kautz, D., Benfield, S., & Carnevale, T. (2008). Evaluation of the Outcome-Present State Test Model as a way to teach clinical reasoning. *Journal of Nursing Education, 47*(8), 337–344. https://doi.org/10.3928/01484834-20080801-01

Boulet, J. R., Murray, D. J., Kras, J., & Woodhouse, J. (2008). Setting performance standards for mannequin-based acute-care scenarios: An examinee-centered approach. *Simulation in Healthcare, 3*(2), 72–81. doi:10.1097/SIH.0b013e31816e39e2

Brodersen, L. D. (2017). Interventions for test anxiety in undergraduate nursing students: An integrative review. *Nursing Education Perspectives, 38*(3), 131–137. https://doi.org/10.1097/01.NEP.0000000000000142

Brodersen, L. D., & Mills, A. C. (2014). A comparison of two nursing program exit exams that predict first-time NCLEX-RN outcome. *CIN: Computers, Informatics, Nursing, 32*(8), 404–412. https://doi.org/10.1097/CIN.0000000000000081

Cant, P., & Cooper, J. (2010). Simulation-based learning in nurse education: A systematic review. *Journal of Advanced Nursing, 66*, 3–15.

Cappelletti, A., Engel, J. K., & Prentice, D. (2014). Systematic review of clinical judgment and reasoning in nursing. *Journal of Nursing Education, 53*(8), 453–458. https://doi.org/10.3928/01484834-0140724-01

Carraccio, C., Englander, R., Gilhooly, J., Mink, R., Hofkosh, D., Barone, M. A., & Holmboe, E. S. (2017). Building a framework of entrustable professional activities, supported by competencies and milestones, to bridge the educational continuum. *Academic Medicine, 92*(3), 324–330. https://doi.org/10.1097/ACM.0000000000001141

Carter, A. G., Creedy, D. K., & Sidebotham, M. (2015). Evaluation of tools used to measure critical thinking development in nursing and midwifery undergraduate students: A systematic review. *Nurse Education Today, 35*(7), 864–874. https://doi.org/10.1016/j.nedt.2015.02.023

Chen, S., Liang, T., Li, M., & Liao, I. (2011). Effects of concept map teaching on students' critical thinking and approach to learning and studying. *Journal of Nursing Education, 50*, 466–469. https://doi.org/10.3928/01484834-20110415-06

Daley, B. J., Morgan, S., & Black, S. B. (2016). Concept maps in nursing education: A historical literature review and research directions. *Journal of Nursing Education, 55*(11), 631–639. https://doi.org/10.3928/01484834-20161011-05

Day, L., Ziehm, S. R., Jessup, M. A., Amedro, P., Dawson-Rose, C., Derouin, A., ... Remen, R. N. (2017). The power of nursing: An innovative course in values clarification and self-discovery. *Journal of Professional Nursing, 33*(4), 267–270. https://doi.org/10.1016/j.profnurs.2017.01.005

DeVellis, R. F. (2016). *Scale development: Theory and applications* (4th ed.). Los Angeles, CA: SAGE Publications.

Gerdeman, J., Lux, K., & Jacko, J. (2013). Using concept mapping to build clinical judgment skills. *Nursing Education in Practice, 13*, 11–17.

Gubrud-Howe, P. (2008). *Development of clinical judgment in nursing students: A learning framework to use in designing and implementing simulated learning experiences* (Doctoral dissertation). Retrieved from ProQuest Dissertations and Theses database. (UMI No. 3343767)

Gul, R. B., & Boman, J. A. (2006). Concept mapping: A strategy for teaching and evaluation in nursing education. *Nurse Education in Practice, 6*, 199–206.

Haladyna, T. M., Downing, S. M., & Rodriguez, M. C. (2002). A review of multiple-choice item-writing guidelines for classroom assessment. *Applied Measurement in Education, 15*(3), 309–333.

Halstead, J. (Ed.). (2007). *Nurse educator competencies: Creating an evidence-based practice for nurse educators*. New York, NY: National League for Nursing.

Harding, M. (2010). Predictability associated with exit examinations: A literature review. *Journal of Nursing Education, 49*(9), 493–497. https://doi.org/10.3928/01484834-20100730-01

Ironside, P. M., & Spurlock, D. R. (2014). Getting serious about building nursing education science. *Journal of Nursing Education, 53*(12), 667–669. https://doi.org/10.3928/01484834-20141118-10

Jensen, R. (2013). Clinical reasoning during simulation: Comparison of student and faculty ratings. *Nurse Education in Practice, 13*, 23–28. doi:10.1016/j.nepr.2012.07.001

Jones-Schenk, J. (2016). Getting to the root of disparities: Social cognition and the affective domain. *Journal of Continuing Education in Nursing, 47*(10), 443–445. https://doi.org/10.3928/00220124-20160920-04

Kane, M. T. (2006). Validation. In R. L. Brennan (Ed.), *Educational measurement* (4th ed.). Portsmouth, NH: Praeger Greenwood Publishing.

Kardong-Edgren, S., Oermann, M., Rizzolo, M. A., & Odom-Maryon, T. (2017). Establishing inter- and intrarater reliability for high-stakes testing using simulation. *Nursing Education Perspectives, 38*, 63–68.

Kavanagh, J. M., & Szweda, C. (2017). A crisis in competency: The strategic and ethical imperative to assessing new graduate nurses' clinical reasoning. *Nursing Education Perspectives*, *38*(2), 57–62. https://doi.org/10.1097/01.NEP.0000000000000112

Lane, S., Raymond, M. R., & Haladyna, T. M. (2016). *Handbook of test development* (2nd ed.). New York, NY: Taylor & Francis.

Lasater, K. (2007). Clinical judgment development: Using simulation to create an assessment rubric. *Journal of Nursing Education*, *46*(11), 496–503.

Lasater, K. (2011). Clinical judgment: The last frontier for evaluation. *Nurse Education in Practice*, *11*(2), 86–92.

Lasater, K., & Nielsen, A. (2009). The influence of concept-based learning activities on students' clinical judgment development. *Journal of Nursing Education*, *48*(8), 441–446.

Liu, O. L., Frankel, L., & Roohr, K. C. (2014). Assessing critical thinking in higher education: Current state and directions for next-generation assessment. *ETS Research Report Series*, *2014*(1), 1–23. https://doi.org/10.1002/ets2.12009

Manetti, W. G. (2015). *Clinical judgement in baccalaureate pre-licensure nursing students* (Doctoral dissertation). Retrieved from ProQuest Dissertations and Theses database. (UMI No. 3701058)

Mariani, B., Cantrell, M. A., Meakim, C., Prieto, P., & Dreifuerst, K. T. (2013). Structured debriefing on students' clinical judgment abilities in simulation. *Clinical Simulation in Nursing Education*, *9*(5), e1-e9. doi:10.1016/j.ecns.2011.11.009

McDonald, M. (2014). *The nurse educator's guide to assessing learning outcomes* (3rd ed.). Burlington, MA: Jones & Bartlett Learning.

Meakim, C., Boese, T., Decker, S., Franklin, A. E., Gloe, D., Lioce, L., & Borum, J. C. (2013). Standards of best practice: Simulation standard I: Terminology. *Clinical Simulation in Nursing*, *9*(6S), S3-S11. http://dx.doi.org/10.1016/j.ecns.2013.04.001.

Messick, S. (1995). Validity of psychological assessment: Validation of inferences from persons' responses and performances as scientific inquiry into score meaning. *American Psychologist*, *50*, 741–749. https://doi.org/http://dx.doi.org/10.1037/0003-066X.50.9.741

Moss, P. A., Girard, B. J., & Haniford, L. C. (2006). Chapter 4: Validity in educational assessment. *Review of Research in Education*, *30*(1), 109–162. https://doi.org/10.3102/0091732X030001109

Nair, G. G., & Stamler, L. L. (2013). A conceptual framework for developing a Critical Thinking Self-Assessment Scale. *Journal of Nursing Education*, *52*(3), 131–138. https://doi.org/10.3928/01484834-20120215-01

National Council of State Boards of Nursing. (2014). The NCSBN national simulation study: A longitudinal, randomized, controlled study replacing clinical hours with simulation in prelicensure nursing education. *Journal of Nursing Regulation*, *5*(2), S3–S40. https://doi.org/10.1016/S2155-8256(15)30062-4

National League for Nursing. (2012a). *NLN fair testing guidelines*. Retrieved from http://www.nln.org/facultyprograms/facultyresources/fairtestingguidelines.pdf

National League for Nursing. (2012b, February). *The fair testing imperative in nursing education*. Retrieved from http://www.nln.org/aboutnln/livingdocuments/pdf/nlnvision_4.pdf

National League for Nursing. (2012c). *The scope of practice for academic nurse educators (2012 Revision)*. Washington, DC: Author.

Oermann, M. H., & Gaberson, K. B. (2014). *Evaluation and testing in nursing education* (4th ed.). New York, NY: Springer.

Oermann, M. H., Saewert, K. J., Charasika, M., & Yarbrough, S. S. (2009). Assessment and grading practices in schools of nursing: National survey findings part I. *Nursing Education Perspectives*, *30*(5), 274–278.

Oermann, M. H., Yarbrough, S. S., Saewert, K. J., Ard, N., & Charasika, M. (2009). Clinical evaluation and grading practices in schools of nursing: National survey findings part II. *Nursing Education Perspectives*, *30*(6), 352–357. doi:10.1043/1536-5026-30.6.352

Pesut, D. J., & Herman, J. (1999). *Clinical reasoning: The art and science of critical and creative thinking*. Albany, NY: Delmar.

Riddell, T. (2007). Critical assumptions: Thinking critically about critical thinking. *Journal of Nursing Education*, 46(3), 121–126.

Romeo, E. M. (2010). Quantitative research on critical thinking and predicting nursing students' NCLEX-RN performance. *Journal of Nursing Education*, 49(7), 378–386.

Rutherford-Hemming, T., Kardong-Edgren, S., Gore, T., Ravert, P., & Rizzolo, M. A. (2014). High-stakes evaluation: Five years later. *Clinical Simulation in Nursing*, 10(12), 605–610. http://dx.doi.org/10.1016/j.ecns.2014.09.009

Sandahl, S. S. (2010). Collaborative testing as a learning strategy in nursing education. *Nursing Education Perspectives*, 31(3), 142–147.

Searing, L. M., & Kooken, W. C. (2016). The relationship between the California Critical Thinking Disposition Inventory and student learning outcomes in baccalaureate nursing students. *Journal of Nursing Education*, 55(4), 224–226. https://doi.org/10.3928/01484834-20160316-08

Shipman, D., Roa, M., Hooten, J., & Wang, Z. (2013). Using the analytic rubric as an evaluation tool in nursing education: The positive and the negative. *Nurse Education Today*, 32(2012), 246–249. doi:10.1016/j.nedt.2011.04.007

Shirrell, D. (2008). Critical thinking as a predictor of success in an associate degree nursing program. *Teaching & Learning in Nursing*, 3(4), 131–136.

Skúladottir, H., & Svavarsdottir, M. (2016). Development and validation of a Clinical Assessment Tool for Nursing Education (CAT-NE). *Nursing Education in Practice*, 20, 31–38.

Spurlock, D. (2006). Do no harm: Progression policies and high-stakes testing in nursing education. *Journal of Nursing Education*, 45(8), 297–302.

Spurlock, D. (2013). The promise and peril of high-stakes tests in nursing education. *Journal of Nursing Regulation*, 4(1), 4–8.

Spurlock, D., & Hunt, L. (2008). A study of the usefulness of the HESI Exit Exam in predicting NCLEX-RN failure. *Journal of Nursing Education*, 47(4), 157–166.

Spurlock, D. R. (2016). Chapter 4: Measuring educational concepts. In B. Patterson & A. Krouse (Eds.). *Scientific inquiry in nursing education: Advancing the science*. Philadelphia, PA: Lippincott.

Spurlock, Jr. D. R., & Hanks, C. (2004). Establishing progression policies with the HESI Exit Examination: A review of the evidence. *Journal of Nursing Education*, 43(12), 539–545. https://doi.org/10.3928/01484834-20041201-07

St-Onge, C., Young, M., Eva, K. W., & Hodges, B. (2017). Validity: One word with a plurality of meanings. *Advances in Health Sciences Education*, 22(4), 853–867. https://doi.org/10.1007/s10459-016-9716-3

Stevens, D., Levi, A., & Walvoord, B. (2012). *Introduction to rubrics: An assessment tool to save grading time, convey effective feedback, and promote student learning* (2nd ed.). Sterling, VA: Stylus Publishing.

Stewart, M. (2011). Joined up thinking? Evaluating the use of concept-mapping to develop complex system learning. *Assessment & Evaluation in Higher Education*, 3, 349–368.

Strickland, H. P., Cheshire, M. H., & March, A. L. (2017). Clinical judgment during simulation: A comparison of student and faculty scores. *Nursing Education Perspectives*, 38(2), 85–86. https://doi.org/10.1097/01.NEP.0000000000000109

Tanner, C. A. (2006). Thinking like a nurse: A research-based model of clinical judgment in nursing. *Journal of Nursing Education*, 45(6), 204–211.

Tanner, C. A. (2011). The critical state of measurement in nursing education research. *Journal of Nursing Education*, 50(9), 491–492. https://doi.org/10.3928/01484834-20110819-01

Tavakol, M., & Dennick, R. (2011). Making sense of Cronbach's alpha. *International Journal of Medical Education*, 2, 53–55. https://doi.org/10.5116/ijme.4dfb.8dfd

Taylor, L. D. (2014). *The affective domain in nursing education: Educators' perspectives*. (Doctoral dissertation). Retrieved from the University of Wisconsin Milwaukee Digital Commons. (Accession No. 109774671).

Thorndike, R. M., & Thorndike-Christ, T. M. (2011). *Measurement and evaluation in psychology and education* (8th ed.). Boston, MA: Pearson.

Valiga, T. M. (2014). Attending to affective domain learning: Essential to prepare the kind of graduates the public needs. *Journal of Nursing Education*, *53*(5), 247. https://doi.org/10.3928/01484834-20140422-10

Walsh, C. M., & Seldomridge, L. A. (2005). Clinical grades: Upward bound. *Journal of Nursing Education*, *44*, 162e–168e.

Walsh, C. M., & Seldomridge, L. A. (2006). Critical thinking: Back to square two. *Journal of Nursing Education*, *45*(6), 212–219.

Ward, T. D. (2015). Do you hear what I hear? The impact of a hearing voices simulation on affective domain attributes in nursing students. *Nursing Education Perspectives*, *36*(5), 329–331. https://doi.org/10.5480/14-1448

Wellmon, R., Lefebvre, K. M., & Ferry, D. (2017). Effects of high-fidelity simulation on physical therapy and nursing students' attitudes toward interprofessional learning and collaboration. *Journal of Nursing Education*, *56*(8), 456–465. https://doi.org/10.3928/01484834-20170712-03

Willhaus, J., Burleson, G., Palaganas, J., & Jeffries, P. (2014). Authoring simulations for high-stakes student evaluation. *Clinical Simulation in Nursing*, *10*(4), e177-e182. http://dx.doi.org/10.1016/j.ecns.2013.11.006

Yeo, C. (2014). Concept mapping: A strategy to improve critical thinking. *Singapore Nursing Journal*, *41*(3), 2–7.

6

Competency IV: Participate in Curriculum Design and Evaluation of Program Outcomes

Martha M. Scheckel, PhD, RN

Jennifer Hedrick-Erickson, MSN, RN, CNL

Nurse faculty are responsible for participating in curriculum design and program evaluation. To do so fully and competently, faculty most often achieve competencies in this area of nursing education through formal degree programs and/or certifications, as well as continuing education opportunities with a focus on curriculum and instruction. As faculty navigate the terrain of curriculum design and program evaluation, it is imperative that they use evidence-based practices from research and standards and guidelines to assist them in enacting this important nursing education skill. Attending to the landscape of contemporary approaches to curriculum design and evaluation ensures students learn within environments that optimally prepare them for practice arenas.

To effectively participate in curriculum design and evaluation of program outcomes, the nurse educator

> ensures that the curriculum reflects institutional philosophy and mission, current nursing and health care trends, and community and societal needs, so as to prepare graduates for practice in a complex, dynamic, multicultural health care environment;

> demonstrates knowledge of curriculum development, including identifying program outcomes, developing competency statements, writing learning objectives, and selecting appropriate learning activities and evaluation strategies;

> bases curriculum design and implementation decisions on sound educational principles, theory, and research;

> revises the curriculum based on assessment of program outcomes, learner needs, and societal and health care trends;

> implements curricular revisions using appropriate change theories and strategies;

> creates and maintains community and clinical partnerships that support educational goals;

> collaborates with external constituencies throughout the process of curriculum revision; and

> designs and implements program assessment models that promote continuous quality improvement in all aspects of the program.

REVIEW OF THE LITERATURE

The literature search for this chapter was conducted using EBSCOhost Academic Search Complete databases: Cumulative Index to Nursing and Allied Health (CINAHL Plus with Full Text), Education Research Complete, Educational Resources Information Center (ERIC), Healthsource: Nursing/Academic Edition, Medline, PsychARTICLES, PsychINFO, and American doctoral dissertations. Broad terms used for the initial search include curriculum design, curriculum evaluation, and program evaluation; applied limiters include 2005–2017, periodical, article, research (when selection available), and the English language. This approach to searching the literature expanded and enriched the literature review for this chapter by including literature from across disciplines, capturing the spirit of interprofessional education.

The literature search yielded 167 results, which were placed in the following themes: addressing trends and issues in health and health care in the curriculum, addressing curriculum delivery methods, integrating simulation into the curriculum, engaging stakeholders in curriculum design, incorporating student input into curriculum design processes, and evaluating program outcomes to ensure continuous quality improvement. The literature was further searched within these themes using the EBSCOhost Academic Search Complete databases that were used for the initial search, and then separately searching for additional literature in databases: PubMed, SAGE Journals, and ScienceDirect. Only research articles were selected for inclusion to ensure that this chapter includes evidence-based literature about curriculum design and program evaluation.

As compared to the evidence-based findings published in Halstead (2007) about curriculum design and program evaluation, there is an increase in curricular intervention studies, which test new curriculum models or processes, and literature syntheses studies (i.e., systematic reviews and integrative reviews), which provide recommendations for best practices in curriculum and evaluation. In addition, this chapter uses the research to formulate statements about what nurse educators should be able to know or do in fulfillment of this competency. What follows is a synthesis of the research literature within the specific themes identified previously. The chapter concludes with a description of gaps in the research and priorities for future research.

Addressing Trends and Issues in Health and Health Care in the Curriculum

Studies about curriculum design conducted from 2005 to 2017 center on the need for faculty to stay current on topics reflecting emerging trends and issues in nursing, the nursing profession, and health and health care. The study designs are diverse and range from descriptive studies to curricular intervention studies. Key topics receiving the most attention published during this time period include genetics, mental health, ethics, and gerontology. Limitations of these research studies lie in the paucity of research designs with high-level evidence (e.g., randomized control trials) and an absence of research in other significant trends and issues such as quality and safety in nursing education. A synthesis of published research (2005-2017) related to these identified topics and what nurse educators should be able to know or do in fulfillment of curriculum design competencies follows.

Genetics

Research about genetics includes descriptive studies in undergraduate and graduate education of faculty, academic administrators', and students' knowledge and perceptions of genetics for the purpose of integrating genetics into curricula (Donnelly, Nersesian, Foronda, Jones, & Belcher, 2017; Edwards, Maradiegue, Seibert, Macri, & Sitzer, 2006; Goldgar & Rackover, 2007; Hsiao, Van Riper, Lee, Chen, & Lin, 2011; Maradiegue, Edwards, Seibert, Macri, & Sitzer, 2005). While the authors of the studies recognized the importance of integrating genetics into the curriculum, they noted a lack of progress in this area that they attributed to a need to increase teachers' self-efficacy in genetics instruction. To address this lack of progress, researchers developed instruments for measuring students' baseline genetic literacy (Bowling et al., 2008; Ward, 2012). Nurse educators can learn to use these evidence-based instruments to increase their competency in assessing student knowledge. They can also seek out faculty development opportunities to increase their ability to integrate genetics concepts into curricula.

Mental Health

Studies about mental health center on descriptive designs that measure undergraduate students' attitudes toward those with mental health disorders to inform ways to minimize bias and stereotypes (Miller, 2017; Schafer, Wood, & Williams, 2011; Surgenor, Dunn, & Horn, 2005). Studies also focus on faculty-practitioner-designed curricular interventions that demonstrate improved preparation of students to care for those with mental health conditions and increased desires to choose careers as mental health care providers (Curtis, 2007; Spence, Garrick, & McKay, 2012). In addition, there is research about including consumers in designing mental health curricula. This research includes (1) a systematic review of consumer involvement in the education of health professionals (Happell et al., 2014); (2) a literature review of consumer participation in designing, developing, and evaluating occupational therapy programs (Arblaster, MacKenzie, & Willis, 2015); (3) a national survey that analyzed nurse academic coordinators' responses to the level and nature of consumer involvement in mental health nursing education (Happell, Platania-Phung, et al., 2015); and (4) a qualitative exploratory study about nurse academics and consumer participation in mental health education for health professionals (Happell, Bennetts, Platania-Phung, & Tohotoa, 2015). These studies suggested benefits of involving consumers in curriculum development, particularly in relation to understanding experiences of those with mental health conditions. However, this research demonstrated that consumer involvement in curriculum design is (1) variable with weak levels of evidence, (2) laden with concerns about vulnerable population involvement in curriculum design, and

(3) replete with concerns about consumers using involvement to express discontent about mental health services. The research about the inclusion of mental health concepts in the curriculum suggests nurse educators must develop competence in addressing students' attitudes toward those with mental health and other health conditions, learn to work with practitioners to develop contemporary curricula, and proceed cautiously, but effectively, to involve consumers in curriculum development.

Ethics

Studies about the effective integration of ethics into the curriculum include those about ethical concepts, utilization of a model core curriculum for teaching medical ethics and law, and use of evidence from critical incidents and program assessment data to integrate ethics into a curriculum. Yazdani, Lakeh, Ahmady, Foroutan, and Afshar (2015) completed a critical interpretive synthesis about the concept of value (i.e., what is considered important) in medical education. Through their analysis, a values-based framework consisting of values' principles, outcomes, and virtues emerged that faculty can use as a resource to guide the integration of the concept of values into the curriculum. McKercher, Mackenzie, Prideaux, and Pang (2014) focused on the concept of social responsibility, comparing attitudes of hospitality and tourism of undergraduate students across 21 economic systems in five continents who had coursework in global environmental issues to students who did not have this coursework. They concluded the coursework made no difference in learner attitudes, leading to the need for faculty to reconsider how to create learning activities that develop students' ethical sense of social responsibility.

Mattick and Bligh (2006) conducted a study of a model core curriculum for teaching medical ethics and law in 22 of 28 medical schools in the United Kingdom. Their purpose was to determine how faculty integrated the core curriculum into medical schools seven years following a consensus statement about the need to use the curriculum model. This study found there was substantial, but not full, integration of the model, suggesting a need for faculty to assess outcomes of integrating standardized core curricula about ethics into a curriculum. Fornari (2006) demonstrated the value of using learning theories and curriculum design concepts to develop a learner-centered, case-based ethics curriculum derived from critical incident evidence (descriptions of clinical events). Similarly, Fossen, Anderson-Meger, and Zellmer (2014) demonstrated how to use program assessment data to devise an ethical decision-making model for infusion into a bachelor of social work curriculum. The compendium of these research studies indicates that nurse educators need to critically evaluate learner outcomes related to including ethical concepts and standardized ethics curricula for the development of students' ethical comportment. Further, faculty need to develop competencies in using evidence to devise approaches for integrating ethics into the curriculum.

Gerontology

Studies about integrating gerontology into the curriculum abound and are situated in the need to prepare health care professionals to care for the growing population of older adults. Much of the research is limited to descriptive studies that identify the extent to which gerontology content is included in the curriculum (Blundell, Gordon, Gladman, &

Masud, 2009; Fagerberg & Gilje, 2007; Harris, 2013). Additionally, studies describe student and faculty attitudes toward caring for older adults (Moone, 2007; Olson, 2007); outcomes of infusing gerontology content into curricula (Lee, Collins, Mahoney, McInnis-Dittrich, & Boucher, 2006); and the impact of training programs to equip educators with the tools they need to include geriatrics in curricula (Masciadrelli, 2014; Mehrotra, Townsend, & Berkman, 2013). These studies point to a need for nurse educators to identify appropriate geriatric curriculum content, understand ways to positively shape student attitudes toward older adults, and learn about faculty development approaches to ensure the teaching of dignified care for this population of patients.

Addressing Curriculum Delivery Methods

Studies about curriculum design also focus on delivery methods, the vehicles through which students engage with curricula. Delivery methods reflecting trends in higher education and documented in the research literature during the time frame associated with this review are problem-based learning, competency-based education, interprofessional education, and the concept-based curriculum. There is a plethora of published research (2005-2017) about these methods with varying levels of evidence, ranging from descriptive studies to systematic reviews. The methods and accompanying evidence help nurse educators make decisions about delivery methods that are congruent with their program's vision, mission, values, and outcomes.

Problem-Based Learning

Introduced nearly 30 years ago, problem-based learning (PBL) arose as a curriculum delivery method that has since been used across disciplines. PBL helps students connect real-life experiences (often through use of case studies) to concepts (O'Neill & Hung, 2010). PBL also allows time for students to discuss topics, which contributes to strong critical thinking skills. O'Neill and Hung (2010) described this critical thinking as students' ability to understand situational knowledge through examining the detail on the "forest floor" (p. 15), while also understanding the broader "landscape" (p. 15) of topics under study. They recommended providing learners with ample resources to enhance the knowledge needed for learning broader contexts.

Research studies supporting PBL as a curriculum delivery method that were published between 2005 and 2017 include Hallinger and Lu's (2012) study in which course evaluation data from 20,988 graduate management students who learned within PBL environments were analyzed over a seven-year time period. Their study suggested how PBL is an active learning strategy favored by students. Another quasi-experimental study of 125 undergraduate business statistics students learning through a conception-focused curriculum (similar to PBL) suggested this type of curriculum increased students' perceptions of being "higher order learners and global citizens" (Burch, Burch, Heller, & Batchelor, 2015, p. 485). The researchers highlighted that utilization of a conception-focused curriculum requires that teachers know how to select discipline-specific concepts and develop learning activities that help students integrate them for understanding disciplinary knowledge. A questionnaire distributed to 60 master of multimedia and technology students over a three-year period indicated that enhancing PBL with various forms of technology, such as Facebook and other digital tools, increased students' satisfaction with learning environments (Ioannou, Vasiliou, & Zaphiris, 2016). However, the researchers pointed out that for PBL to be effective, faculty must know how to facilitate the social and cognitive components of this delivery method.

Given these studies and the understandings derived from the long history of PBL, the nurse educator will find relevance in using it as a curriculum delivery method. Students enjoy learning from real-world examples that are easily and immediately applicable. However, the nurse educator must embrace PBL as an active learning method and be willing to engage in faculty development to know how to use PBL and various modalities to deliver PBL (e.g., through concepts or using technology). In addition, faculty must be cognizant of PBL's limitations. They must ensure that students avoid the study of particular situations devoid of the theories underpinning broader contexts.

Competency-Based Education

Another curriculum delivery method populating the literature is competency-based education (CBE). In existence since the late 19th century, CBE experienced a resurgence in the 1970s and is now enjoying a revival due to political climates promoting efficient and cost-effective educational models (Gallagher, 2014). Competency-based education was modeled after K-12's mastery learning (Nodine, 2016). It allows students to progress at their own pace once they demonstrate mastery of particular knowledge, skills, and attitudes. This delivery method is widely cited throughout the literature as a curriculum framework for medical students.

Gruppen et al. (2016) related that CBE focuses on curricular outcomes, strengthens students' abilities, reduces training time, and encourages learner involvement. Research regarding the use of CBE is sparse and, in part, supports Gruppens's statement regarding the nature of CBE. Fastré, van der Klink, Amsing-Smit, and van Merriënboer (2014), who used an experimental design to study competency-based and performance-based education for stoma care skills, demonstrated that learning outcomes are enhanced through combining competency-based and performance-based education (e.g., evaluating students on the task [performance] *and* the ability to perform the task well [competency]).

Simonds, Behrens, and Holzbauer (2017) compared use of CBE in an online and in-classroom introductory psychology course, and showed that with either format, CBE increased students' ownership of learning and their ability to transfer learning to other contexts. However, they reported that educators must invest time to learn CBE and formally orient students to the methodology so they understand its applications to learning. The research literature about CBE, therefore, indicates that nurse educators who want to use this curriculum delivery approach would benefit from reviewing the research published in medical education literature, combine it with other curriculum delivery methods for robust impact on learner outcomes, and engage in faculty development for effective implementation.

Interprofessional Education

Another trend in curriculum delivery methods is interprofessional education (IPE), "when students from two or more professions learn about, from and with each other to enable effective collaboration and improve health outcomes" (World Health Organization, 2010, p. 7). Speakman (2016) conveys that implementing IPE is challenging because it is difficult to determine learning experiences and appropriately time them in curricula.

To address these challenges, Loversidge and Demb (2015) conducted a phenomenological study of nursing and medical faculty. Their purpose was to interpret and understand experiences of curricula and pedagogies they use to help students learn IPE and what hinders and removes barriers to IPE. The findings suggested that faculty want IPE to provide "authentic experiences" (p. 300), which include debriefing and narrative reflection. The researchers expressed the need for administration to make IPE a priority and involve all faculty in IPE, including adjunct faculty.

Rajamani, Westra, Monsen, LaVenture, and Gatewood (2015), on the other hand, focused on academic-practice partnerships to address challenges in implementing IPE, using a case study research method to examine interprofessionalism and informatics. Their work resulted in the "Minnesota Framework for Interprofessional Biomedical Health Informatics," which highlights how education and practice partners can collaborate to ensure they meet one another's outcomes while being attuned to future trends. Importantly, they underscored the need for students to understand the roles of professions other than their own, and how to work effectively as a team. The limited studies addressing faculty competencies for implementing IPE indicate that IPE will be most effective if faculty know how to seek and obtain broad faculty and administrative support. Facilitating academic-practice partnerships is suggested as a mechanism for implementation.

Concept-Based Curriculum

The concept-based curriculum (CBC) is another trend in the research about curriculum delivery methods. As compared to other research, studies about CBC have most frequently been in nursing education as a mechanism for preventing content saturation. When aptly implemented, CBC is student centered, encourages critical thinking, and helps students understand concepts as opposed to memorizing content (Giddens et al., 2008; Giddens, Wright, & Gray, 2012). The CBC research in nursing education is limited to single-site studies; however, the findings of this research show promise in relation to how CBC improves students' critical thinking skills.

Gooder and Cantwell (2017) developed and administered a survey and conducted focus groups to measure students' perceptions of CBC. Forty-one associate degree nursing students and 54 RN-BSN completion students completed the survey, with 8 students participating in the focus groups. The researchers found that students were satisfied or completely satisfied with CBC and reported that it helped them think critically, rather than simply memorize and regurgitate content. Patterson, Crager, Farmer, Epps, and Schuessler (2016) compared three classes that were taught using CBC; they found it improved students' critical thinking skills and that faculty and clinical facilities were positive about its impact on critical thinking.

Likewise, Sportsman and Pleasant (2017) conducted two surveys (one in 2014 and one in 2016) to elicit information from nursing education administrators about the efficacy of CBC. They also conducted focus groups to identify experiences about development and implementation. They found that students in a CBC curriculum demonstrated better clinical judgment than students being taught in a more traditionally delivered curriculum.

Despite the research on CBC, a barrier to implementation is faculty members' lack of knowledge about the approach, the time it takes for faculty to learn it, and their fear of losing "role identity" (Hendricks & Wangerin, 2017, p. 141). Hendricks and Wangerin suggested the loss of role identity is related to the CBC requirement for faculty to work in teams to thread concepts across the curriculum, which may threaten their autonomy over content expertise. To this end, nurse educators using CBC must undergo faculty development to effectively facilitate its implementation. They must embrace CBC as a faculty-faculty collaborative effort in overcoming content saturation in nursing education.

Engaging Stakeholders in Curriculum Design

Much of the research about curriculum design addresses the need to engage stakeholders from the outset as a means of facilitating congruence between education and practice. In this way, stakeholders become partners with academic institutions, collaborating with them to revise curricula, rather than observers of change, with limited opportunities to provide nursing programs with feedback (Keogh, Fourie, Watson, & Gay, 2010).

The research about involving stakeholders is limited to qualitative studies and centered *on only stakeholders* and their role in curriculum design *or* stakeholders and their role in multifaceted curriculum change processes. Within these studies, the definition of stakeholder varies. It is as narrow as teachers and students or as broad as teachers, students, patients, clinicians, community partners, and organizations associated with educational programs. The purpose of the curriculum redesign often facilitates decision-making about who is identified as a stakeholder and the extent of the stakeholder's involvement in the changes taking place.

With regard to research focusing on only stakeholders, one study examined stakeholder involvement in learning about, assessing, identifying, and delineating key skills (e.g., communication, information technology, working with others) for a midwifery curriculum (Dixon & Donovan, 2004). Another identified the need to use a learning community concept to develop a curriculum for clinical educators that focused on educational theory and teaching practices (McAllister & Moyle, 2006). In addition, Keogh et al. (2010) explicated the experiences of being a stakeholder in developing a new undergraduate nursing curriculum. They found that stakeholder involvement created a collective sense of ownership of the curriculum.

In relationship to engaging stakeholders within a multifaceted change process, Johnson et al. (2007) described a study in which a literature review and interviews with stakeholders resulted in goal statements outlining needs to ensure that future dental school curricula address oral health disparities. Similarly, McCallum (2008) used case study methodology to analyze data from document reviews, interviews, and surveys of health care providers and medically underserved adult stakeholders to design a curriculum with a service-learning orientation.

Nosek, Scheckel, Waterbury, MacDonald, and Wozney (2017) described a study in which the Collaborative Improvement Model (Waterbury, 2010) facilitated stakeholder involvement in workgroups charged with specific tasks in preparing to revise an undergraduate nursing curriculum (e.g., analyze external guidelines, review past and present program data, complete curriculum mapping, and identify best practices). The findings of their study suggested the process bridged disparate cultures within two campuses and promoted the scholarship of teaching and learning.

The studies about stakeholder involvement in curriculum design support stakeholder contributions in facilitating novel and robust approaches to curriculum change and integration into the academic community. The evidence thus suggests that nurse educators must recognize the need for and value of involving stakeholders in curriculum change processes. Educators must also draw on evidence for direction about how to identify stakeholders that are important to curriculum change, develop skills in collaboration to devise ways to involve them in curriculum change, and focus on how to ensure ethical and judicious use of stakeholders' contributions to the curriculum change process.

Obtaining Student Input into Curriculum Design Processes

Several studies focus on obtaining student input into curriculum design processes. The emphasis on student input originates from the recent trend away from a teacher-centered educational philosophy to a student- or learner-centered philosophy. A learner-centered philosophy presupposes that, through teaching, students become motivated and empowered to have control over their learning (Weimer, 2013). In relation to soliciting student input into curriculum design, Bovill (2014) used a case study methodology and critical theory to examine faculty members' experiences at three universities cocreating curricula in the fields of geography, education, and environmental justice. Bovill's study demonstrated that a learner-centered philosophy increases students' responsibility for learning and enhances their performance while also increasing teachers' satisfaction as they learn from students.

Studies of student input into curriculum design fell into two categories in which students provided (1) input as part of curriculum redesign processes and (2) feedback before and/or after curriculum redesign processes. Research about input into curriculum redesign included the use of focus groups with students on how to include health systems sciences (HSS) in a medical school's curriculum (Gonzalo, Haidet, Blatt, & Wolpaw, 2016). Analysis of data from the focus groups revealed that curricula were "trapped in an education world where students' focus is dominated by exams, clerkship performance and residency vetting, which largely ignore the importance of HSS" (p. 528). The authors suggested using Kegan and Lahey's (2009) immunity-to-change approach to change the unchangeable toward promoting HSS. This approach offers an important method for educators to challenge and change "sacred cows" when redesigning curricula.

Two additional studies recommended that faculty use action research to engage students in curriculum change. McCuddy, Pinar, and Gingerich (2008) applied action-research-oriented organizational development and change (ODC) to obtain diagnostic data from students to change a business school curriculum. The ODC process included surveying students and conducting focus groups to identify students' perceptions and insights about the curriculum. The result was meaningful action to change the curriculum. O'Neill and McMahon (2012) suggested a similar approach to ODC when they implemented a participatory research and action (PRA) approach as a mechanism for including the voices of undergraduate physiotherapy students in initiating curriculum changes. In their study, students created pie charts of curriculum issues, participated in plenary whole-class curriculum discussions, and provided solutions to curriculum issues. The authors indicated that when faculty used PRA, they empowered students to be involved in curriculum changes and strengthened their voice in the process.

Two studies that provided feedback before and/or after curriculum redesign used a pre- and posttest design. One study measured geriatric competencies for the purpose of building a learner-centered geriatric curriculum for medical students (McCrystle, Murray, & Pinheiro, 2010). Another validated a creative curriculum innovation for culinary students (Hu, Horng, & Teng, 2016). A third study used a participatory action research design where patients provided data to measure students' caring behaviors following implementation of a caring course within a caring curriculum in an associate degree nursing program (Lee-Hsieh, Kuo, Turton, Hsu, & Chu, 2007). Each of these studies yielded positive findings in relation to faculty use of student-based data to informing curriculum redesign.

Studies of student input into curriculum design suggest that nurse educators should juxtapose principles, theoretical frameworks, and inductive research methods with student input for curriculum change (e.g., applying immunity to change principles, using ODC, using participatory action research methods). The literature also highlights the value of nurse educators gathering pre- and/or posttest data from students about curriculum changes to guide rigorous, learner-centered curriculum redesign.

Evaluating Program Outcomes to Ensure Continuous Quality Improvement

Overall, the research about evaluating program outcomes to ensure continuous quality improvement is sparse and limited by single-site studies. Nonetheless, the research encompasses important new trends that include the involvement of stakeholders in program evaluation. This trend aligns with the "Engaging Stakeholders in Curriculum Design" theme previously described. Linnan et al. (2010) described a benchmarking study conducted in a master of public health degree program, which included an analysis of benchmarks of program requirements at 11 peer institutions, juxtaposing those findings with surveys of stakeholder groups about their program. Findings resulted in recommendations for changes ranging from improving advising and mentoring to increasing elective credit offerings.

Morris and Hancock (2013) engaged stakeholders (described as nursing student consumers of nursing programs and faculty) using a mixed-methods approach. They triangulated data from the Institute of Medicine's (IOM) core competencies, a course objectives matrix, data from student and faculty surveys of perceptions about integration of IOM competencies into the curriculum, and open-ended questions to evaluate the integration of the IOM's competencies into the curriculum. Their findings suggest a need for faculty to be intentional about designing learning experiences that facilitate implementing the IOM competencies (e.g., revise objectives to directly reflect the competencies). Studies suggest that the nurse educator's ability to involve stakeholders in program evaluation methods for continuous quality improvement fosters the generation of knowledge that can be used for program improvement efforts.

IDENTIFIED GAPS IN THE LITERATURE

The evidence-based review of literature conducted for this chapter illuminates what nurse educators need to be able to know or do (i.e., competencies) to participate in curriculum design and the evaluation of program outcomes. These competencies are informed through research studies that, as compared to the chapter on this core competency in Halstead (2007), remain somewhat sparse. However, the studies described in this chapter do represent research designs that offer stronger evidence than in the previous publication. For example, the current review includes more systematic reviews. This changing landscape of study designs is encouraging and points to a need for conducting studies designed to generate a strong body of research to contribute to evidence-based nursing education.

In comparing the research to the task statements, the evidence suggests continued emphasis on health care trends that mirror community and society needs. However, the research for this task statement falls short in its emphasis on understanding multiculturalism within these trends. There is also good evidence around using sound principles, theory, and research to design curricula, especially in the area of curriculum delivery where "tried and true" methods dominate—methods that have been used for decades (e.g., problem-based learning). The evidence is also strong about the need to create and maintain clinical partnerships that support educational goals and collaborate with external constituencies throughout the process of curriculum revision. Studies such as those involving consumers in the design of mental health curricula, engaging in academic-practice partnerships for interprofessional education, and using stakeholder involvement and student input into curriculum design are some of the many ways in which nursing education is expanding its borders to facilitate the development of a curriculum that is tied to the "real world."

Despite these strengths in the research, there is very little research to help educators with best practices in the task statement pertaining to identifying program outcomes, developing competency statements, writing learning objectives, and selecting appropriate learning activities and evaluation strategies. The research does measure learning outcomes as evidence for the extent to which a curriculum design approach was effective, but there is little research directly linked to this competency. The same gap exists for the task statement about designing and implementing program assessment models that promote continuous quality. Very little research is available to assist nurse educators in developing evidence-based competencies in this area, leaving a large void in what is a critical part of the optimal operations of a nursing program.

In addition, the use of change theories and strategies, central to any curriculum redesign undertaking, is virtually absent, with the exception of studies about student input into curriculum design. Finally, noticeably absent from the literature are research studies focused on graduate education curriculum design and program evaluation, as most studies were conducted in undergraduate education, and faculty development studies to demonstrate how to facilitate the transition from practice to academics, particularly in the area of curriculum development and evaluation, for the novice educator.

PRIORITIES FOR FUTURE RESEARCH

In light of the gaps in the research described previously, and as compared to the evidence-based findings published in Halstead (2007) about curriculum design and program evaluation, the following priorities for research mirror those needed over 10 years ago:

> What are best practices for attaining educator competencies in identifying program outcomes, developing competency statements, writing learning objectives, and selecting appropriate learning activities and evaluation strategies?

> What are best practices for attaining educator competencies in designing and implementing program assessment models that promote continuous quality?

> What are best practices for attaining educator competencies in the use of change theories and strategies for curriculum redesign and program evaluation?

In addition to priorities that remain, new priorities have become apparent from this review of the literature. These priorities highlight gaps while building on emerging areas of research:

> What study designs about curriculum redesign and program evaluation could encompass multiculturalism?

> What study designs are needed to determine how to most effectively integrate stakeholder involvement into traditional program evaluation models to produce best practices in continuous quality improvement?

> What competencies do faculty need to ensure that graduate education has a source of best practices?

> What are best approaches for faculty development for novice educators in curriculum design and program evaluation?

References

Arblaster, K., Mackenzie, L., & Willis, K. (2015). Mental health consumer participation in education: A structured literature review. *Australian Occupational Therapy Journal, 62*(5), 341–362. doi:10.1111/1440-1630.12205

Blundell, A., Gordon, A., Gladman, J., & Masud, T. (2009). Undergraduate teaching in geriatric medicine: The role of national curricula. *Gerontology & Geriatrics Education, 30*(1), 75–88. doi:10.1080/02701960802690324

Bovill, C. (2014). An investigation of co-created curricula within higher education in the UK, Ireland and the USA. *Innovations in Education and Teaching International, 51*(1), 15–25. doi:10.1080/14703297.2013.770264

Bowling, B. V., Acra, E. E., Wang, L., Myers, M. F., Dean, G. E., Markle, G. C., ... Huether, C. A. (2008). Development and evaluation of a genetics literacy assessment instrument of undergraduates. *Genetics, 178*(1), 15–22. doi:10.1534/genetics.107.079533

Burch, G. F., Burch, J. J., Heller, N. A., & Batchelor, J. H. (2015). An empirical investigation of the conception focused curriculum: The importance of introducing undergraduate business statistics students to the "real world." *Decision Sciences Journal of Innovative Education, 13*(3), 485–512. doi:10.1111/dsji.12074

Curtis, J. (2007). Working together: A joint initiative between academics and clinicians to prepare undergraduate nursing students to work in mental health settings. *International Journal of Mental Health Nursing, 16*(4), 285–293. doi:10.1111/j.1447-0349.2007.00478.x

Dixon, A., & Donovan, P. (2004). Implementation of a key skills agenda within an undergraduate programme of midwifery studies. *Nursing Education Today, 24*(6), 483–490.

Donnelly, M. K., Nersesian, P. V., Foronda, C., Jones, E. L., & Belcher A. E. (2017). Nurse faculty knowledge of and confidence in teaching genetics/genomics: Implications for faculty development. *Nurse*

Educator, 42(2), 100–104. doi:10.1097/
NNE.0000000000000297

Edwards, Q. T., Maradiegue, A., Seibert,
D., Macri, C., & Sitzer, L. (2006). Faculty
members' perceptions of medical genetics
and its integration into nurse practitioner
curricula. *Journal of Nursing Education,
45*(3), 124–130.

Fagerberg, I., & Gilje, F. (2007). A comparison
of curricular approaches of care of the
aged in Swedish and US nursing programs.
Nurse Education in Practice, 7(6), 358–364.
doi:10.1016/j.nepr.2006.11.007

Fastré, G. J., van der Klink, M. R., Amsing-
Smit, P., & van Merriënboer, J. G. (2014).
Assessment criteria for competency-based
education: A study in nursing education.
Instructional Science, 42(6), 971–994.
doi:10.1007/s11251-014-9326-5

Fornari, A. (2006). Developing an ethics curriculum using learner-centered pedagogy.
*International Journal of Allied Health Sci-
ences and Practice, 4*(2), 1–6.

Fossen, C., Anderson-Meger, J., & Zellmer,
D. A. D. (2014). Infusing a new ethical
decision-making model throughout a BSW
curriculum. *Journal of Social Work Values
and Ethics, 11*(1), 66–81.

Gallagher, C. W. (2014). Disrupting the game-
changer: Remembering the history of
competency-based education. *Change, 46*(6),
16–23. doi:10.1080/00091383.2014.969177

Giddens, J., Brady, D., Brown, P., Wright, M.,
Smith, D., & Harris, J. (2008). A new
curriculum for a new era of nursing education. *Nursing Education Perspectives, 29*(4),
200–204.

Giddens, J. F., Wright, M., & Gray, I. (2012).
Selecting concepts for a concept-based
curriculum: Application of a benchmark
approach. *Journal of Nursing Education,
51*(9), 511–515. doi:10.3928/014834-
20120730-02

Goldgar, C., & Rackover, M. (2007). Current
status of genetics education and needs
assessment of physician assistant programs: A national survey. *Journal of Physician Assistant Education, 18*(2), 53–59.

Gonzalo, J. D., Haidet, P., Blatt, B., & Wolpaw,
D. R. (2016). Exploring challenges in

implementing a health systems science
curriculum: A qualitative analysis of student perceptions. *Medical Education, 50*,
523–531. doi:10.1111/medu.12957

Gooder, V., & Cantwell, S. (2017). Student
experiences with a newly developed concept-based curriculum. *Teaching & Learning
in Nursing, 12*(2), 142–147. doi:10.1016/j.
teln.2016.11.002

Gruppen, L. D., Burkhardt, J. C., Fitzgerald,
J. T., Funnell, M., Haftel, H. M., Lypson, M.
L., ... Vasquez, J. A. (2016). Competency-
based education: Programme design and
challenges to implementation. *Medical
Education, 50*(5), 532–539. doi:10.1111/
medu.12977

Hallinger, P., & Lu, J. (2012). Overcoming the
Walmart syndrome: Adapting problem-
based management education in East Asia.
*Interdisciplinary Journal of Problem-Based
Learning, 6*(1), 16–42. doi:10.7771/1541-
5015.1311

Halstead, J. (Ed). (2007). *Nurse educator
competencies: Creating an evidence-based
practice for nurse educators.* New York:
National League for Nursing.

Happell, B., Bennetts, W., Platania-Phung, C.,
& Tohotoa, J. (2015). Consumer involvement
in mental health education for health professionals: Feasibility and support for the
role. *Journal of Clinical Nursing, 24*(23-24),
3584–3593. doi:10.1111/jocn.12957

Happell, B., Byrne, L., McAllister, M., Roper,
C., Gaskin, C. J., Martine, G., ... Hamer, H.
(2014). Consumer involvement in tertiary-
level education of mental health professionals: A systematic review. *International
Journal of Mental Health Nursing, 23*(1),
3–16. doi:10.1111/inm.12021

Happell, B., Platania-Phung, C., Byrne, L.,
Wynaden, D., Martiarris, S., & Harris, S.
(2015). Consumer participation in nurse
education: A national survey of Australian
universities. *International Journal of Mental
Health Nursing, 24*(2), 95–103. DOI:
10.1111/inm.12111

Harris, L. J. (2013). *A case study of Connecticut
community college nursing programs to describe gerontological content inclusion in associate degree registered nursing programs*

using an education curriculum framework (Doctoral dissertation, University of Hartford, CT). Retrieved from http://digitalcommons.goodwin.edu/cgi/viewcontent.cgi?article=1000&context=nursing_fac_pubs

Hendricks, S. M., & Wangerin, V. (2017). Concept-based curriculum: Changing attitudes and overcoming barriers. *Nurse Educator, 42*(3), 138–142. doi:10.1097/NNE.0000000000000335

Hsiao, C. Y., Van Riper, M., Lee, S. H., Chen, S. J., & Lin, S. C. (2011). Taiwanese nursing students' perceived knowledge and clinical comfort with genetics. *Journal of Nursing Scholarship, 43*(2), 125–132. doi:10.1111/j.1547-5069.2011.01389.x.

Hu, M., Horng, J., & Teng, C. (2016). Developing a model for an innovative culinary competency curriculum and examining its effects on students' performance. *Journal of Creative Behavior, 50*(3), 193–202. doi:10.1002/jocb.139

Ioannou, A., Vasiliou, C., & Zaphiris, P. (2016). Problem-based learning in multimodal learning environments: Learners' technology adoption experiences. *Journal of Computing Research, 54*(7), 1022–1040. doi:10.1177/0735633116636755

Johnson, B. R., Loomer, P. M., Siegel, S. C., Pilcher, E. S., Leigh, J. E., Gillespie, J., ... Turner, S. P. (2007). Strategic partnerships between academic dental institutions and communities: Addressing disparities in oral health. *Journal of the American Dental Association, 138*(10), 1366–1371. doi:10.14219/jada.archive.2007.0054

Kegan, R., & Lahey, L. L. (2009). *Immunity to change: How to overcome it and unlock the potential in yourself and your organization.* Boston, MA: Harvard Business Press.

Keogh, J. J., Fourie, W. J., Watson, S., & Gay, H. (2010). Involving stakeholders in the curriculum process: A recipe for success. *Nurse Education Today, 30*(1), 37–43. doi:10.1016/j.nedt.2009.05.017

Lee, E., Collins, P., Mahoney, K., McInnis-Dittrich, K., & Boucher, E. (2006). Enhancing social work practice with older adults: The role of infusing gerontology content into the master of social

work foundation curriculum. *Educational Gerontology, 32*(9), 737–756. doi:10.1080/03601270600835454

Lee-Hsieh, J., Kuo, C., Turton, M. A., Hsu, C., & Chu, H. (2007). Action research on the development of a caring curriculum in Taiwan: Part II. *Journal of Nursing Education, 46*(12), 553–561.

Linnan, L. A., Steckler, A., Maman, S., Ellenson, M., French, E., Blanchard, L., ... Moracco, B. (2010). Engaging key stakeholders to assess and improve the professional preparation of MPH health educators. *American Journal of Public Health, 100*(10), 1993–1999. doi:10.2105/AJPH.2009.177709

Loversidge, J., & Demb, A. (2015). Faculty perceptions of key factors in interprofessional education. *Journal of Interprofessional Care, 29*(4), 298–304. doi:10.3109/13561820.2014.991912

Maradiegue, A., Edwards, Q. T., Seibert, D., Macri, C., & Sitzer, L. (2005). Knowledge, perceptions, and attitudes of advanced practice nursing students regarding medical genetics. *Journal of the American Academy of Nurse Practitioners, 17*(11), 472–479. doi:10.1111/j.1745-7599.2005.00076.x

Masciadrelli, B. P. (2014). "I learned that the aging population isn't that much different from me": The final outcomes of a Gero-Ed BEL Project. *Journal of Gerontological Social Work, 57*(1), 24–36. doi:10.1080/01634372.2013.854855

Mattick, K., & Bligh, J. (2006). Undergraduate ethics teaching: Revisiting the consensus statement. *Medical Education, 40*(4), 329–332. doi:10.1111/j.1365-2929.2006.02407.x

McAllister, M., & Moyle, W. (2006). Stakeholders' views in relation to curriculum development approaches for Australian clinical educators. *Australian Journal of Advanced Nursing, 24*(2), 16–20.

McCallum, C. (2008). A process of curriculum development: Meeting the needs of a community and a professional physical therapist education program. *Journal of Physical Therapy Education, 22*(2), 18–28.

McCrystle, S. W., Murray, L. M., & Pinheiro, S. O. (2010). Designing a learner-centered geriatrics curriculum for multilevel medical learners. *Journal of the American Geriatrics Society*, *58*, 142–151. doi:10.1111/j.1532-5415.2009.02663.x

McCuddy, M. K., Pinar, M., & Gingerich, E. F. R. (2008). Using student feedback in designing a student-focused curricula. *International Journal of Educational Management*, *22*, 611–637. doi:10.1108/09513540810908548

McKercher, B., Mackenzie, M., Prideaux, B., & Pang, S. (2014). Is the hospitality and tourism curriculum effective in teaching personal social responsibility? *Journal of Hospitality & Tourism Research*, *38*(4), 431–462. doi:10.1177/1096348012451452

Mehrotra, C. M., Townsend, A., & Berkman, B. (2013). Evaluation of a training program in aging research for social work faculty. *Educational Gerontology*, *39*(11), 787–796. doi:10.1080/03601277.2012.734155

Miller, R. (2017). Australian undergraduate nursing students' opinions on mental illness. *Australia Journal of Advanced Nursing*, *34*(3), 34–42. doi:10.4103/0253-7176.140701

Moone, R. (2007). Aging at the University of Minnesota's School of Social Work: Historiography of gerontological curriculum. *Educational Gerontology*, *33*(11), 955–967. doi:10.1080/03601270701631885

Morris, T. L., & Hancock, D. R. (2013). Institute of Medicine core competencies as a foundation for nursing program evaluation. *Nursing Education Perspectives*, *34*(1), 29–33.

Nodine, T. R. (2016). How did we get here? A brief history of competency-based higher education in the United States. *Journal of Competency Based Education*, *1*(1), 5–11. doi:10.1002/cbe2.1004

Nosek, C. M., Scheckel, M. M., Waterbury, T., MacDonald, A., & Wozney, N. (2017). The collaborative improvement model: An interpretive study of revising a curriculum. *Journal of Professional Nursing*, *33*(1), 38–50. doi:10.1016/j.profnurs.2016.05.006

Olson, M. D. (2007). Gerontology content in MSW curricula and student attitudes toward older adults. *Educational Gerontology*, *33*(11), 981–994. doi:10.1080/03601270701632230

O'Neill, G., & Hung, W. (2010). Seeing the landscape and the forest floor: Changes made to improve the connectivity of concepts in a hybrid problem-based learning curriculum. *Teaching in Higher Education*, *15*(1), 15–27. doi:10.1080/13562510903488006

O'Neill, G., & McMahon, S. (2012). Giving student groups a stronger voice: Using participatory research and action (PRA) to initiate change to a curriculum. *Innovations in Education and Teaching International*, *49*(2), 161–171. doi:10.1080/14703297.2012.677656

Patterson, L. D., Crager, J. M., Farmer, A., Epps, C. D., & Schuessler, J. B. (2016). A strategy to ensure faculty engagement when assessing a concept-based curriculum. *Journal of Nursing Education*, *55*(8), 467–470. doi:10.3928/01484834-20160715-09

Rajamani, S., Westra, B. L., Monsen, K. A., LaVenture, M., & Gatewood, L. C. (2015). Partnership to promote interprofessional education and practice for population and public health informatics: A case study. *Journal of Interprofessional Care*, *29*(6), 555–561. doi:10.3109/13561820.2015.1029067

Simonds, J., Behrens, E., & Holzbauer, J. (2017). Competency-based education in a traditional higher education setting: A case study of an introduction to psychology course. *International Journal of Teaching & Learning in Higher Education*, *29*(2), 412–428.

Speakman, E. (2016). Interprofessional education and collaborative practice. In D. M. Billings, & J. A. Halstead (Eds.), *Teaching in nursing: A guide for faculty* (5th ed., pp. 186–196). St. Louis, MO: Elsevier.

Spence, D., Garrick, H., & McKay, M. (2012). Rebuilding the foundations: Major renovations to the mental health component of an undergraduate nursing curriculum. *International Journal of Mental Health Nursing*, *21*(5), 409–418. doi:10.1111/j.1447-0349.2011.00806.x

Sportsman, S., & Pleasant, T. (2017). Concept-based curricula: State of the innovation. *Teaching & Learning in Nursing*, *12*(3), 195–200. doi:10.1016/j.teln.2017.03.001

Surgenor, L. J., Dunn, J., & Horn, J. (2005). Nursing student attitudes to psychiatric nursing and psychiatric disorders in New Zealand. *International Journal of Mental Health Nursing, 14*(2), 103–108. doi:10.1111/j.1440-0979.2005.00366.x

Ward, L. D. (2012). *Development of the genomic nursing concept inventory* (Unpublished doctoral dissertation, Washington State University).

Waterbury, T. (2010). Using the collaborative improvement model to improve a university hiring process. *International Journal Productivity & Quality Management, 5*(1), 75–87.

Weimer, M. (2013). *Learner-centered teaching: Five key changes to practice* (2nd ed.). San Francisco, CA: Jossey-Bass.

World Health Organization. (2010). *Framework for action on interprofessional education & collaborative practice*. Retrieved from http://hsc.unm.edu/ipe/resources/who-framework-.pdf

Yazdani, S., Lakeh, M. A., Ahmady, S., Foroutan, A., & Afshar, L. (2015). Critical interpretive synthesis of the concept of value in medical education. *Research & Development in Medical Education, 4*(1), 31–34. doi:10.15171/rdme.2015.005

7

Competency V: Function as a Change Agent and Leader

Jennifer A. Specht, PhD, RN
Dawn M. Gordon, PhD, MS, MBA, RN, PHN

In addition to preparing graduates who practice effectively and thrive in complex health care environments, contemporary nurse educators are charged with acting as and developing nurse leaders who use their voices to advocate for the nursing profession and for quality patient care. Nurse educators function as change agents and advocates to strengthen the voice of nursing and nursing education. Today's health care climate necessitates a strong nursing presence that comes from the empowerment afforded by solid educational foundations and perspectives. It is the responsibility of nurse educators to bolster their own leadership skills, as well as those of undergraduate and graduate students, through formal and informal education. Ideally, the leadership competencies and examples exemplified by nurse educators not only model leadership skills for learners but also empower nurse graduates to act as future change agents in the profession. To be successful advocates for change, nurse educators need to develop their leadership competencies, as well as their personal leadership style.

Nurse educators effect change in the nursing profession through their personal leadership contributions and by empowering their students and graduates to become leaders. Leadership in nursing is necessary for the advancement of nursing practice, education, and science. In addition to the impact of their own leadership platforms, which include programmatic improvement, scholarship, and political activism, nurse educators have a unique opportunity to teach and develop leadership abilities among their students. The current state of health care necessitates innovative approaches to teaching and learning to educate nurses who are prepared to be competent practitioners and advocates for the nursing profession and patients.

Attention to developing future nurse leaders is imperative for the meaningful expansion of nursing leadership in the various capacities needed in nursing and health care. Therefore, it is essential that nurse educators advance their own leadership skills and abilities and develop key competencies as leaders and change agents to shape the future of the nursing profession and effectively impart leadership abilities to their students. Ideally nurse educators will have benefited from a solid undergraduate experience related to leadership and received support and mentoring throughout their careers to strengthen their leadership capabilities. Gazza & Sterrett (2011) outlined strategies for planning and engaging in a successful leadership journey, noting that the nurse educator's "leadership journey begins during undergraduate education and extends throughout the career continuum" (p. 59).

Nursing education plays a central role in shaping the quality of leadership in the United States by setting curricular standards, determining who will educate future leaders (Outcalt, Faris, McMahon, & Astin, 2001), and emphasizing that leadership involves engagement via speaking up and being visible (Hofmeyer, Sheingold, Klopper, & Warland, 2015). The development of nurses who are empowered to use their voices and skills to act as future change agents necessitates the incorporation of leadership competencies into curricular design and rigorous educational experiences.

To successfully sculpt future leaders, it is essential for nurse educators to develop themselves as leaders in nursing and to teach and role model leadership skills and characteristics (Grossman & Valiga, 2005) that will, in turn, embolden graduates to use their voices to impact change in nursing and health care. Nurses' voices blend their knowledge and expertise with a perspective focused on the holistic patient to advocate for patient-centered practices and policies. The influential voices of leaders in nursing cultivate collaboration between nursing education and practice, as well as interprofessional collaboration that leads to safe, effective, and quality patient care (Cox, Cuff, Brandt, Reeves, & Zierlere, 2016; Institute of Medicine [IOM], 2015). In their function as change agents and leaders in nursing, nurse educators create a preferred future for nursing education and nursing practice.

Nursing education is foundational to the development of leaders who will serve to support a strong nursing presence that will positively impact patient care and inform and influence health care policy. The National League for Nursing's (NLN's) Excellence in Nursing Education Model (2006a) outlines eight core elements necessary to achieve and sustain excellence in nursing. Two key elements are inclusive of the need for leadership: well-prepared faculty and student-centered, interactive, and innovative programs and curricula.

The need for well-prepared faculty encompasses academic leaders, as well as expert researchers and clinicians. Academic leadership focuses on the advancement of the profession, mentoring of faculty, advisement of students related to career development, teaching and evaluation of individual students, and program assessment and evaluation. According to the NLN Excellence in Nursing Education Model (2006a), a key aspect of well-prepared faculty is the charge to provide leadership to transform and re-vision nursing education. This emphasizes the importance of leadership development in nurse educators and ultimately the graduates of nursing programs.

Designing student-centered, interactive, and innovative programs and curricula, as referenced in the NLN's Excellence in Nursing Education Model (2006a), also includes the integration of leadership competencies. It is clear from this model that leadership is an essential component of excellence in nursing education that extends to nursing practice and quality patient care. To demonstrate competence as a change agent and leader, a nurse educator.

› models cultural sensitivity when advocating for change;

› integrates a long-term, innovative, and creative perspective into the nurse educator role;

> participates in interdisciplinary efforts to address health care and educational needs locally, regionally, nationally, or internationally;

> evaluates organizational effectiveness in nursing education;

> implements strategies for organizational change;

> provides leadership in the parent institution and in the nursing program to enhance the visibility of nursing and its contributions to the academic community;

> promotes innovative practices in educational environments; and

> develops leadership skills to shape and implement change.

REVIEW OF THE LITERATURE

Over the last decade, there has been a marked expansion of the evidence-based literature related to leadership in nursing education and nursing. This expansion of leadership-related literature provides much-needed insight into nursing leadership competencies that must be developed in, and by, nurse educators. The foundational approaches necessary to strengthen the voice and presence of nursing within the governing structures of academic communities and health care systems, as well as regional, national, and international communities, is now better understood.

There are multiple ways for nurse leaders to effect change in nursing education, nursing practice, and health care as a whole. Leadership in nursing is broad based and inclusive of titled and nontitled leadership roles. Titled roles include dean and program director, hospital administrator, and elected officer and director of professional organizations, among others. Of equal importance are the nontitled leaders in nursing who contribute to the advancement of nursing or nursing education through research, activism, or professional expertise. Both types of leaders are needed to strengthen and sustain the voice of nursing that is necessary to advocate for patients and for the nursing profession. With today's health care environment experiencing unprecedented growth and reformation, requiring solid leadership to appropriately transform organizational values, beliefs, processes, and behaviors (Wolf, Triolo, & Ponte, 2008), fostering leadership, beginning at the undergraduate level, is essential to long-term and profound effects on the quality of health care.

The evidence for this review related to leadership in nursing was gleaned from approximately 15 evidence-based publications, various other scholarly resources, and professional organization statements and guidelines. Databases such as Cumulative Index to Nursing and Allied Health Literature (CINAHL), Education Resources Information Center (ERIC), and EBSCOhost were searched for publications for the period 2005 through 2017. Studies were sought for review using keywords such as change agents, leaders, leadership, nursing education, nursing, nursing administration, and faculty. Qualitative, quantitative, and mixed-methods study designs, as well as systematic reviews, were prioritized. Relevant reports and white papers, conceptual frameworks, literature reviews, and books were used to gather and expand upon concepts and key findings. Searches were not inclusive of dissertations or theses, but international publications were included.

Evidence-based literature related to the leadership of nurse educators prior to 2005 identified themes of leading and managing change in education systems and developing leadership styles and skills. These two general themes have been expanded upon as additional concepts have emerged. The more recent literature (2005–2017) is focused on better defining key characteristics and competencies of nurse educators related to leadership (Davidson, Weberg, Porter-O'Grady, & Malloch, 2017; Patterson & Krouse, 2015) and on broadening and providing rationale for priorities for leaders in nursing. There are multiple avenues through which nurse educators can effect change through leadership (Grossman & Valiga, 2017; McBride, 2011) and an identified need to focus on developing future leaders in our nursing students (Barry, Houghton, & Warburton, 2016; Grossman & Valiga, 2017). Nurse educators, students, and graduates with savvy leadership abilities and strong voices are respected in educational and health care system settings, professional associations, and public-political arenas. The vision for leadership in nursing is ultimately focused on value-based, quality, affordable, and equally inclusive health care. The major themes in the literature related to leadership in nursing education for the period 2005 to 2017 are (1) advancing personal leadership potential, (2) organizational success and change, (3) collaboration for best practices, and (4) advocacy for change.

Advancing Personal Leadership Potential

Developing leadership characteristics and skills in nurses has been a key topic in education and practice alike. Leadership abilities can be learned and developed, and leaders can emerge and evolve through education, experiences, and purposeful effort (Grossman & Valiga, 2017). In their cross-sectional, online survey of faculty and administrators at top nursing schools in the United States, Delgado and Mitchell (2016) reported that 78 percent of respondents believed that academic leadership can be learned. Leadership development is a priority for organizations such as the NLN as evident in their offering of formal leadership development programs. The NLN Leadership Institute, which encompasses the Leadership Development for Simulation Educators, LEAD, and Executive Leadership in Nursing Education and Practice programs, encourages participants to enhance their personal and professional leadership development (NLN, 2017).

Twenty-one nurse faculty leaders interviewed by Young, Pearsall, Stiles, Nelson, and Horton-Deutsch (2011) described their experiences as leaders, and three themes emerged: feeling as though they were thrust into leadership, taking risks, and learning to face challenges. Given the findings that nurse faculty leaders felt underprepared for leadership positions, formal preparation that supports and encourages leadership development, through coursework or mentoring, was recommended.

Delgado and Mitchell's (2016) survey of 52 nurse educators and academic nursing leaders identified integrity, clarity in communication, and problem-solving ability as the qualities most important for academic leaders in nursing; a track record in research was the least important quality. More than half of the respondents (53.1 percent) reported participating in leadership development beyond their basic nursing preparation; 78.8 percent of them believed participation made a difference. The most common types of leadership development opportunities in which respondents participated were mentoring, which was highly valued, and on-the-job training. Respondents also developed their leadership competencies by attending leadership classes in graduate programs and formal leadership programs within and external to their places of employment. The results from Delgado and Mitchell's study suggest that lifetime learning and foundational knowledge are the basis for leadership development in the face of the "serious challenges that are unique to our times: a paucity of qualified faculty, competition for other resources, and continual and rapid technological and social changes" (p. 15). Their work is evidence that personal leadership development, as well as organizational support and investment, is needed to develop leaders in nursing.

Leadership in nursing education bolsters the collective voice of nursing in higher education, as well as in the health care arena. The constant changes in health care delivery drive priorities for leadership and practice in nursing education. Patterson and Krouse (2015) interviewed 15 leaders in nursing education related to their thoughts surrounding the essential competencies that nurse educators need to be leaders in nursing education. The researchers found four competencies: articulate and promote a vision for nursing education, function as a steward for the organization and nursing education, embrace professional values in the context of higher education, and develop and nurture relationships. The identification of these key competencies informs the development of leaders in nursing through nursing education by embracing and strengthening the impact of nurse educators. Relationships with disciplines outside of nursing within educational institutions help to enrich perspectives related to clinical concepts, cultivate interdisciplinary collaboration, and improve appreciation of the foci of other professions. Relationships with key players in health care systems, as well as holding leadership positions within the systems, expand nurse leaders' understanding of the business of nursing.

Leaders in nursing function to advance the profession through significant contributions that have an impact now and in the future. Acquiring and continuing to improve one's leadership skills are essential aspects of professional nursing, for both nurse educators and clinical nurses. Nurse educators, in addition to developing and exercising their personal leadership abilities, need to integrate leadership course content into the curricula of all programs and role model leadership behaviors in their teaching roles. Grossman and Valiga (2017) purport nurse educators should foster leadership in their students by helping them integrate leadership as an integral component of their roles; their focus should be as much on the development of leadership skills as on the acquisition of clinical skills. Benner, Sutphen, Leonard, and Day (2010) describe a call to action for educating nursing students to become agents of change to influence political and public arenas to improve health care systems. Nurse educators, they say, must focus on teaching students to embrace their authority, not just their responsibility, to practice nursing.

In addition to role modeling leadership behaviors, nurse educators need to engage in mentoring relationships that foster leadership development in both faculty and students. Mentoring relationships in nursing education can decrease role conflict and ambiguity in junior nurse educators (Specht, 2013) and can serve to foster overall faculty development and build leadership potential (Delgado & Mitchell, 2016). Through mentoring relationships, nurse educators can gain exposure to opportunities that enable them to impact change by utilizing their leadership abilities in their home institutions and in various external venues.

As leaders, nurse educators can influence processes and policies within educational institutions, health care systems, and professional organizations. For example, Grossman and Valiga (2005) charged leaders to be actively involved in professional organizations as a means to advocate for positive change in nursing and health care. Nurse researchers also act as change agents by creating and disseminating knowledge that informs education and practice. As nurse educators expand their leadership abilities and integrate leadership behaviors and roles into their professional identities, they can simultaneously be mentees and mentors for peers, students, and other developing leaders.

Mentoring relationships help build the leadership pipeline by supporting future leaders in nursing (Branden & Sharts-Hopko, 2017). A cycle of mentoring, while being mentored in nursing education, can bolster leadership abilities in faculty and provide insight and guidance to students, allowing them to integrate leadership into their practice. Beyond curricula, nursing education is a platform for teaching leadership characteristics through role modeling and mentoring. Leadership theory taught in the classroom needs demonstration and reinforcement in clinical and real-world settings to facilitate student learning and the development of leadership skills (Barry et al., 2016). Garrity (2013) found reflective journaling to be an effective teaching strategy to increase a learner's critical thinking and the application of new knowledge related to leadership.

To be effective change agents, and to teach others leadership skills, leaders in nursing need to develop effectual leadership styles. Many variables influence leadership style and how nurses lead change in the complex and continually changing nursing environment. McBride (2011) highlights nursing leadership styles and the applications of situational decisions or tensions that guide the nursing profession. Her key tenets are leadership as personal, leadership as achieving organization goals, and leadership as transformational. McBride challenges effective leaders to expand their thinking and develop new skills to meet organizational missions and specific goal achievements.

The concept of transformational leadership is prevalent in nursing research and is suggested as a method to champion for organizational and workplace cultures of safety (IOM, 2004). The American Nurses Credentialing Center's (2011) Magnet Recognition Program identifies the quality of nursing leadership as one of the major forces determining health care system quality. In its Magnet Model, the center specifically distinguishes transformational leadership related to global issues in nursing and health care. Some research suggests transformational leadership is a primary tenet of nursing leadership and change (Marshall & Broome, 2017). Merrill (2015) explored the relationship between nurse manager leadership styles and safety climates of 41 nursing departments across nine hospitals. Study findings indicated transformational leadership was a positive contributor to safety climates, while laissez-faire leadership style was a negative contributor to unit socialization and a culture of blame. Nurse leaders need to be aware of staff nurse perceptions of positive and negative leadership styles to promote safety and success within organizations. Brewer et al. (2016) researched transformational leadership and found it to create a positive work environment that supports nurses, with the potential to slow attrition and retain nurses. The situational application of appropriate types of leadership styles influences safety and organizational success.

Organizational Success and Change

Solidification of leadership skills and a firm understanding of one's personal leadership style can enhance the ability to recognize and evaluate organizational strengths and weaknesses. Nurse leaders' understanding of current priorities in both education and health care systems can broaden their perspectives and allow for the development of a symbiotic relationship among organizations. An understanding of organizational dynamics allows leaders in nursing to have a positive influence on organizational processes and bring about improvements in nursing education, educational institutions, and health care systems. To effectively and collectively transform health care, all nurses need to integrate leadership skills as a vital component of their professional roles (Grossman & Valiga, 2017).

Promoting effective leaders is a primary objective of top health care systems. Thus, educational institutions continue to prioritize leadership research and development in hopes of building a more robust nursing workforce. As leaders in nursing, nurse educators promote a vision of nursing education while functioning as stewards for organizations by developing relationships and embracing professional values in the context of higher education (Patterson & Krouse, 2015). Nurse leaders work to bridge gaps in communication and establish relationships between educational institutions and health care systems to positively affect graduate preparation with the ultimate goal of improving patient outcomes while containing costs. The evolution of this synergistic dialogue can serve the mission and goals of the educational institution and the health care system and translate into more viability for both types of organizations. The thoughtful and purposeful application of leadership style can lead to effective planning, streamlining of processes, and operationalization of organizational vision.

Innovations and organizational transformations can be successful when developed in the right context of leadership style, skills and behaviors, and timing balance. Martin, McCormack, Fitzsimons, and Spirig (2014) interviewed nurse leaders and conducted focus group interviews with the leaders and their teams to determine the benefits of a shared vision as an essential feature of leadership behavior. The researchers identified vision as key to achieving a shared goal when energies are focused and balanced appropriately within a systematic process for evaluation. The findings encourage leaders in nursing to focus on core values that are realistic and achievable to meet organizational vision. Inspiration and commitment to the vision are enacted from strong leadership skills, attributes, and awareness.

The American Organization of Nurse Executives (AONE, 2015) published competencies about five leadership domains that are critical for both educational institutions and health care system success. These domains are communication and relationship building, knowledge of the health care environment, leadership skills, professionalism, and business skills. AONE notes that the work environment for nurses, in both clinical and academic settings, is important for their satisfaction and retention, and ultimately the success of the organization.

The Nursing Organizations Alliance (NOA, 2004) established nine principles and elements of healthy work environments that support the notions of communicative and collaborative practice, competent and visible leadership, continued professional development, and recognition of the value of nursing's contribution to practice. The NLN, recognizing these elements as having implications in the academic work setting, developed the Healthful Work Environment Tool Kit (NLN, 2006b), to be used to evaluate and to create, or continually improve upon, a healthy work environment as one that enables faculty to provide quality nursing education. Leadership is identified as one of the areas critical to healthy work environments, and the NLN's tool kit offers questions exploring institutional leadership, as well as resources related to leadership. Leaders in nursing, in particular nurse administrators, are very influential in determining the overall health of the work environment and, fundamentally, the culture of the organization (Brady, 2010). Organizationally attuned and visible leaders are key to organizational success. A health care system's likelihood for success is often attributed to nursing leadership.

O'Connor and Carlson (2016) focused on the development of leadership skills to promote a positive impact on clinical nursing staff and enhance a culture of safety. Their study, which reviewed a community hospital's culture and leadership development, found that senior leaders created strong ties with clinical staff. The researchers identified the significant attributes of a successful culture as communication, advocacy, visibility, and access to leaders in nursing. Leaders in nursing recognize the need for and create organizational change leading to better processes and outcomes. The complexity and fluidity of today's health care arena necessitate nurses who embody leadership in nursing and health care to improve patient access to care. According to Grossman and Valiga (2017), it is important that nursing care be recognized as the reason for positive and cost-effective patient outcomes.

Organizational success can be enhanced by establishing a culture that encourages leadership development and supports potential leaders in nursing. Wong and colleagues' (2013) national Canadian study explored bedside nurses' interests in formal management roles and the factors affecting their decision-making by conducting 18 focus groups with 125 staff nurses and managers. Among the major themes and subthemes influencing nurses' decisions to pursue management roles were personal disposition, with a subtheme of leadership skills, and situation, with the subthemes of leadership development opportunities, manager role perceptions, and presence of mentors. Wong and colleagues' findings pointed to an organizational need to provide support and leadership development and succession opportunities, and to redesign manager roles for optimum success. An organizational culture that supports leadership development and potential leaders is equally important in educational institutions. Adams (2007) surveyed nursing academic administrators and full-time faculty of 54 accredited nursing programs in the United States related to the shortage of qualified candidates interested in academic nursing administration. She found that 63 percent of full-time faculty at the participating institutions would not consider moving into positions with greater administrative responsibility.

Young et al. (2011) raised additional concerns when their interviews of 21 nurse educators revealed that participants were in unsought and unanticipated roles as leaders in academia for which they felt unprepared. They found nurse educators currently in leadership roles within educational institutions who did not wish to be in the roles and/or had minimal or insufficient leadership education. Siddique, Aslam, Khan, and Fatima (2011), in their exploration of the concepts of academic leadership, motivation of faculty members, and organizational effectiveness, suggested that decreased investment and engagement in nursing administrative roles can lead to decreased faculty satisfaction and retention. Leaders in nursing are essential to creating the change necessary to support those currently in, or potentially interested in, leadership roles. The leadership pipeline must be strengthened by leaders in nursing through succession planning and mentoring of those interested in leadership roles. This proactive approach to leadership development is the stewardship necessary to optimize the long-term success of organizations (Branden & Sharts-Hopko, 2017).

Organizational administrative structure is also important for the effectiveness and sustainability of nursing education programs and institutions of higher learning, as well as health care systems. Administrative structure should not only maximize organizational efficiency and outcomes but also support leadership development. In their cross-sectional correlational survey of 519 registered nurses in the Netherlands, Knol and Van Linge (2009) found that, to support a culture that encourages the empowerment of nurses, organizations need to create an organizational structure that promotes both formal and informal power. In their systematic review of the relationship between structural empowerment and psychological empowerment for registered nurses, Wagner et al. (2010) purported that providing structural empowerment in an environment is an important organizational strategy to create positive work behaviors and attitudes. Optimizing the organizational structure of administrative roles should be tailored to current and future needs, as well as the needs of patients and staff, or faculty and students.

Nurse educators can bolster leadership development in students that may empower graduates to take on both titled and nontitled leadership roles in their practice, whether in nursing education programs, institutions of higher learning, or health care systems. Regan et al. (2017) explored the perspectives of 42 new graduate nurses and 28 unit nurse leaders regarding new graduate nurses' transition experiences in Canadian health care settings. Their descriptive qualitative study used inductive content analysis of focus groups and interview data from new graduate nurses and unit nurse leaders to identify common factors that facilitate transition into practice. The factors they identified include formal orientation programs, unit cultures that encourage constructive feedback, and supportive mentors. Regan et al. found barriers to successful transition into practice, including unanticipated changes to orientation length, inadequate staffing, uncivil unit cultures, and heavy workloads. The findings support incorporating leadership development into nursing programs, and the use of role modeling and mentoring relationships that can foster the growth of students and new graduates.

Nurse educators can broaden their leadership abilities by exposing themselves to the business side of nursing and by engaging with other disciplines within their educational institutions or health care systems. An understanding of external perspectives and priorities can be gleaned by formally serving on committees or task groups or by participating in interdisciplinary research or initiatives, or informally through relationships with other members of educational institutions or health care systems. This not only develops faculty but also forges relationships among nursing programs and key affiliates, leading to a more comprehensive perspective and optimal success. This perspective can be shared with students in the classroom and through role modeling.

Collaboration for Best Practice

Leadership in nursing, regardless of whether the setting is in education or practice, brings people together to accomplish the common goal of quality patient care. In their textbook related to transformational leadership, Marshall and Broome (2017) provide a review of collaborative projects in which nurses had opportunities to work with multidisciplinary leaders inside and outside a workplace or organization. The nurses and leaders, together in collegial relationships, offered each other new perspectives and renewed energy. Together they developed professional relationships and networks, created connections, and forged partnerships.

Nurse leaders create and work toward shared visions to effect change and achieve quality patient care (Grossman & Valiga, 2017). In addition to facilitating collaboration between nursing education and practice, leaders stimulate change through interprofessional collaboration, leading to safe, effective, and quality patient care. In two published reports, the IOM touted how essential nurse leaders are to the health of the United States in the 21st century. The 2004 IOM report, *Keeping Patients Safe,* identified transformational leadership as a means to promote organizational and workplace cultures of safety. The 2011 IOM report, *The Future of Nursing: Leading Change, Advancing Health,* charges nurses to act as full partners with physicians and other health care professionals for safe and effective care. The report challenges nurses to work to the full scope of their practice and to contribute to the redesign of health care in the United States within a collaborative team. Grossman and Valiga (2017) concur that today's health care arena necessitates that leaders in nursing be involved in multidisciplinary collaboration.

Collaborative practice and achieving cost-effective, quality patient outcomes are at the forefront of health care research and development. Interprofessional education (IPE) has been a platform for educational and practice initiatives that have stimulated change in nursing and nursing leadership. The Interprofessional Education Collaborative (IPEC), aspiring to develop interprofessional competencies of health profession students as part of the learning process, published the *Core Competencies for Interprofessional Collaborative Practice* report (IPEC, 2011). The report details several frameworks reflecting the need for communication, and for the unification of priorities, between health profession programs, including nursing, and health care systems. The frameworks offer schematics that explain the interdependence between health professions' education and practice needs, and reflect the call for leadership. The role of nursing in IPE and collaborative practice is essential for safe, effective, and quality care. Zwarenstein, Goldman, and Reeves (2009) stressed that research focused on interprofessional practice and related health care outcomes exists but is currently limited and unable to generalize key elements of interprofessional practice and its effectiveness. Research on the value of interprofessional collaboration on actual patient outcomes is a next step for real-world application in leading nursing change.

As stated previously, nurse leaders are essential to the achievement of quality patient care, and nurse educators have the responsibility to foster the development of leadership competencies in their students. The Quality and Safety Education for Nurses (QSEN) institute identified competencies that should be developed during prelicensure nursing education so graduates have the competencies required to work continuously toward improving the quality and safety of health care systems (Cronenwett et al., 2007). Nurses are called to assume leadership roles as part of the necessary knowledge, skills, and attitudes (KSAs) for successful teamwork and collaboration as identified by QSEN. Leadership skills can help nurses function effectively within nursing and interprofessional teams, fostering open communication, mutual respect, and shared decision-making to achieve quality patient care.

To best allow for nurse leaders to impact organizational success and change, they need to be aware of self-care, including how to avoid nurse leader fatigue. There is a growing body of quantitative and qualitative research that raises awareness about the reduction and prevention of nurse leader fatigue. Steege, Pinekenstein, Arsenault Knudsen, and Rainbow (2017) researched nurse managers and executives in a mixed-methods study of 21 hospital nurse administrators. They found that a high prevalence of nurse leader fatigue has the potential to impact turnover intent of nurse administrators and, eventually, quality of care. Consequences of nurse leader fatigue include an impact on decision-making ability, life-work balance, and turnover intention of leaders. Results of the Steege et al. study showcase the significance of programs and policies necessary to prevent nurse leader fatigue and retain essential nurse leaders in our current health care system. A focus on organizational success and the care of leaders in nursing are imperative criteria for the future of nursing leadership.

Advocacy for Change

Leaders in nursing are often pioneers, using foresight and visionary thinking to create the preferred future of nursing. New opportunities arise in practice and education wherever a culture of advocacy for others is supported, allowing nurse leaders to champion positive changes related to nursing and health care. It is necessary for nurse leaders to position themselves and their colleagues so their informed voices are heard among internal and external networks of key players, legislators, and political groups. The voices of leaders in nursing are instrumental in the development of health policy, changing the delivery of health care to consumers through board and committee membership, and taking on leadership positions in policymaking organizations (Grossman & Valiga, 2017; Marshall & Broome, 2017).

A 2009 Gallup (2010) poll of more than 1,500 university faculty, insurance, corporate, health services, government, and industry thought leaders examined views about leadership in nursing and goals for the role of nursing in the future. Opinion leaders viewed nurses as having a great deal of impact on the meaningful elements included in health care reform, but did not see nurses as having a great deal of influence on health care reform. The poll results offered suggestions as to how nurses can increase their influence in key areas of health care and health policy. The message was that nurses need to make their voices heard. Further, the opinion leaders felt nurses are responsible not only for providing quality patient care but also for health care leadership.

Leaders in nursing with strong and informed voices are needed to transform health care. All nurses, in education and in practice, are called to make contributions for the betterment of care delivery. The IOM's 2011 report on the future of nursing encourages nurses to embrace their roles in redesigning and leading changes in health care, including working to influence policy. Currently, nurses are not often well recognized as advocates and leaders of policy change and may be left out of important political discussions. Educational preparation in terms of nurses feeling empowered and authorized to advocate in the political arena is often limited, focusing too much on clinical education instead of policy involvement (Marshall & Broome, 2017). Leaders in nursing offer valuable perspectives on balancing the business of health care with improved patient outcomes. Serving on governing boards of professional or health care organizations, institutes, or similar associations is an essential avenue through which nurses, as leaders, can participate in decisions that directly impact the quality and safety of patient care. Nurses in leadership positions on governing boards, serving as partners with other health care professionals, guide health care system change and demonstrate accountability for their own contributions for the delivery of high-quality care (Pennsylvania Action Coalition, 2017). The national Campaign for Action and state-level action coalitions enhance and highlight this call for action and nudge forward the future work of nurses on boards within their communities and states, as well as nationally (Campaign for Action, 2017).

The world of education has presented some newer challenges to nurse leaders. In ever-evolving nursing programs, leaders are asked to be regulatory managers, create accountability and cost efficiencies, and sustain institutional policy that drives innovation (Patterson & Krouse, 2015). Institutional-level policies are often driven by state and other regulatory or accrediting agencies, reinforcing the need for leaders in nursing education to understand the importance of using their voices to vitally impact policy and governance. Clark, Miller, Leuning, and Baumgartner (2017) explored how nursing education can be a place to practice civic agency to create meaningful changes in health care. This exploration encouraged a curricular focus that promotes the application of nursing leadership skills for participation in public and political discussions related to health care, emphasizing the importance of civic engagement. Students participated in a yearlong project as they became citizen nurses, learning and analyzing skills needed to be effective agents of change. Nurse educators can stimulate civic change through pedagogy utilizing innovative leadership and teaching styles.

Quality leaders need risk-taking skills (Glazer & Fitzpatrick, 2013) to evaluate and calculate the benefit and challenges of risks when serving as advocates for others. At times, nurses take care of the most vulnerable, or those who cannot speak for themselves. The duty of nurse leaders is no different; they hold the power and knowledge to know when the vulnerable or underserved need nurse advocates to champion their health care needs. Leadership involves teaching others to recognize these needs and modeling cultural sensitivity and respect while advocating for vulnerable populations and/or those with health disparities. Nurses guide change by being politically astute and using their power wisely (Glazer & Fitzpatrick, 2013) to support all aspects of population health. The preferred future of nursing is in the hands of nursing leaders who take action, risk choices, and serve their communities, state, or nation to serve those that need our advocacy.

Summary

Effective nurse educators masterfully apply leadership styles and have the necessary skills to drive policy and practice changes, while educating and supporting students and/or staff to ultimately achieve quality patient outcomes. To be successful leaders and change agents, nurse educators have the responsibility to strengthen and retain their leadership competencies in a rapidly changing health care arena. Nurse educators have a pivotal role in the development of nurses who can function effectively and competently in today's health care systems, acting as leaders and promoting the development of future leaders in nursing. To effect positive change in nursing and health care, it is imperative that nurse educators possess the competencies necessary to not only develop leadership skills in their graduates but also inspire graduate voices. Through nursing research and ingenious pedagogy and practice, leaders in nursing influence education, policy, and practice in nursing and health care. Nurses need to be ready and poised to make changes for the preferred future of nursing.

IDENTIFIED GAPS IN THE LITERATURE

This review of the literature provides insight into the foundational competencies and approaches that nurse educators need to strengthen the voice and presence of nursing within the governing structures of academic communities, health care systems, and regional, national, and international communities. Leaders in nursing advance nursing practice, education, and science through their personal leadership initiatives, as well as by developing future leaders in nursing. The last decade has broadened the evidence base related to leadership in nursing education and nursing practice, and its potential impact on health care. Key characteristics and competencies of nurse educators related to leadership, and the priorities for leaders in nursing, have been examined. The need for nurse educators to not only embody leadership in their own professional practice but also develop leadership competencies in students so that they are empowered and authorized to lead has become apparent.

While progress has been made in terms of understanding nurse educators' roles in functioning as change agents and leaders, there are gaps to fill with future inquiry. Exploration of the impact of relationships and partnerships suggested for the stewardship of nursing education, as well as that of mentoring relationships related to leadership potential, is lacking. The need to investigate ways to effectively build the pipeline of leaders in nursing education and practice, and for succession planning, is also evident. Building a more robust future nursing workforce and the promotion of organizational success of nursing programs, educational institutions, and health care systems have been studied, but there is a need for continued research about how to most effectively develop a nursing workforce designed to meet and advocate for the health care needs of patients. Overall, the current research literature reveals some descriptive and qualitative studies that have laid the groundwork to build on these areas of inquiry, but further development in these areas is necessary.

Continued research related to leadership styles, and the situational application of appropriate types of styles, can grow knowledge and guide change for current and future leaders in nursing. Future studies on successes and limitations of interprofessional practice and education would benefit the nursing profession and could serve to expand existing knowledge and positively affect future educational and nursing practice. Further exploration of nurse leader fatigue to best identify awareness, prevention, and reduction of key nursing challenges is an additional gap in a recently growing nursing research area. A body of knowledge supporting the importance of nursing's civic duty exists, but given the current state of health care, further exploration into how leaders in nursing should advocate for others is warranted. Future research is needed to prepare nurses who can function as change agents and leaders in nursing in the various capacities needed in nursing and health care.

PRIORITIES FOR FUTURE RESEARCH

The following questions are offered to stimulate research that will enhance our understanding of the nurse educator competency of functioning as a change agent and leader:

▸ What are the most effective methods for the implementation and evaluation of leadership development in nursing curricula and formal leadership programs?

▸ What are the best practices for providing opportunities for students to be mentored by leaders in nursing inside and outside of educational institutions and health care systems?

▸ How can nursing leaders and organizations support and sustain a leadership pipeline to provide for succession planning in educational institutions, health care systems, and professional nursing organizations?

▸ What are the best collaborative practices for interprofessional education and practice, as well as for building relationships between nursing programs, educational institutions, and health care systems?

▸ What are the most impactful ways to emphasize the variety of roles through which leaders in nursing can effect change in nursing and health care?

▸ How can leaders in nursing affect population health related to vulnerable populations and/or those with health disparities especially in underrepresented areas such as in rural health?

References

Adams, L. (2007). Nursing academic administration: Who will take on the challenge? *Journal of Professional Nursing, 23*(5), 309–315.

American Nurses Credentialing Center. (2011). *Magnet Recognition Program® overview*. Retrieved from http://nursecredentialing.org/Documents/Magnet/MagOverview-92011.pdf

American Organization of Nurse Executives. (2015). *AONE Nurse Executive Competencies*. Chicago, IL: Author. Retrieved from http://www.aone.org/resources/nurse-leader-competencies.shtml

Barry, D., Houghton, T., & Warburton, T. (2016). Supporting students in practice: Leadership. *Nursing Standard, 31*(4), 46–53. doi:10.7748/ns.2016.e9669

Benner, P., Sutphen, M., Leonard, V., & Day, L. (2010). *Educating nurses: A call for radical transformation*. San Francisco, CA: Jossey-Bass.

Branden, P., & Sharts-Hopko, N. C. (2017). Growing clinical and academic nursing leaders: Building the pipeline. *Nursing Administration Quarterly, 41*(3), 258–265. doi:10.1097/NAQ.0000000000000239

Brady, M. (2010). Healthy nursing academic work environments. *Online Journal of Issues in Nursing, 15*(1), Manuscript 6. doi:10.3912/OJIN.Vol15No01Man06

Brewer, C. S., Kovner, C. T., Djukic, M., Fatehi, F., Greene, W., Chacko, T. P., & Yang, Y. (2016). Impact of transformational leadership on nurse work outcomes. *Journal of Advanced Nursing, 72*(11), 2879–2893. doi:10.1111/jan.13055

Campaign for Action. (2017, August 11). *State Action Coalitions*. Retrieved from https://campaignforaction.org/our-network/state-action-coalitions/

Clark, K. M., Miller, J. P., Leuning, C., & Baumgartner, K. (2017). The citizen nurse: An educational innovation for change. *Journal of Nursing Education, 56*(4), 247–250. doi:10.3928/01484834-20170323-12.

Cox, M., Cuff, P., Brandt, B., Reeves, S., & Zierlere, B. (2016). Measuring the impact of interprofessional education on collaborative practice and patient outcomes. *Journal of Interprofessional Care, 30*(1), 1–3. doi:10.3109/13561820.2015.1111052

Cronenwett, L., Sherwood, G., Barnsteiner, J., Disch, J., Johnson, J., Mitchell, P., … Warren, J. (2007). Quality and safety education for nurses. *Nursing Outlook, 55*(3), 122–131.

Davidson, S., Weberg, D., Porter-O'Grady, T., & Malloch, K. (2017). *Leadership for evidence-based innovation in nursing and health professions*. Burlington, MA: Jones & Bartlett Learning.

Delgado, C., & Mitchell, M. M. (2016). A survey of current valued academic leadership qualities in nursing. *Nursing Education Perspectives, 37*(1), 10–15. doi:10.5480/14-1496

Gallup. (2010). *Nursing leadership from bedside to boardroom: Opinion leaders' perceptions*. Princeton, NJ: Robert Wood Johnson Foundation. Retrieved from https://www.rwjf.org/content/dam/farm/reports/reports/2010/rwjf53344

Garrity, M. K. (2013). Developing nursing leadership skills through reflective journaling: A nursing professor's personal reflection. *Reflective Practice, 14*(1), 118–130. doi:10.1080/14623943.2012.732940

Gazza, E. A., & Sterrett, S. E. (2011). The leadership journey: From belief to reality. *Teaching and Learning in Nursing, 6*, 59–63. doi:10.1016/j.teln.2010.10.002

Glazer, G., & Fitzpatrick, J. J. (2013). *Nursing leadership: From the outside in*. New York, NY: Springer.

Grossman, S., & Valiga, T. M. (2005). *The new leadership challenge: Creating the future of nursing* (2nd ed.). Philadelphia, PA: F.A. Davis.

Grossman, S., & Valiga, T. M. (2017). *The new leadership challenge: Creating the future of nursing* (5th ed.). Philadelphia, PA: F.A. Davis.

Hofmeyer, A., Sheingold, B. H., Klopper, H. C., & Warland, J. (2015). Leadership in learning and teaching in higher education: Perspectives of academics in non-formal leadership roles. *Contemporary Issues in Education Research, 8*(3), 181–192.

Institute of Medicine. (2004). *Keeping patients safe: Transforming the work environment of nurses*. Retrieved from http://www.nap.edu/catalog/10851.html

Institute of Medicine. (2011). *The future of nursing: Leading change, advancing health*. Washington, DC: National Academies Press.

Institute of Medicine. (2015). *Measuring the impact of interprofessional education on collaborative practice and patient outcomes*. Washington, DC: National Academies Press.

Interprofessional Education Collaborative. (2011). *Core competencies for interprofessional collaborative practice: Report of an expert panel*. Retrieved from http://www.aacn.nche.edu/education-resources/ipecreport.pdf

Knol, J., & Van Linge, R. (2009). Innovative behaviour: The effect of structural and psychological empowerment on nurses. *Journal of Advanced Nursing, 65*, 359–370. doi:10.1111/j.1365-2648.2008.04876.x

Marshall, E. S., & Broome, M. E. (2017). *Transformational leadership in nursing: From expert clinician to influential leader*. New York, NY: Springer.

Martin, J., McCormack, B., Fitzsimons, D., & Spirig, R. (2014). The importance of inspiring a shared vision. *International Practice Development Journal, 4*(2), 1–15.

McBride, A. B. (2011). *The growth and development of nurse leaders*. New York, NY: Springer.

Merrill, K. C. (2015). Leadership style and patient safety. *Journal of Nursing Administration, 45*(6), 319–324. doi:10.1097/NNA.0000000000000207

National League for Nursing. (2006a). *Excellence in nursing education model*. New York, NY: Author.

National League for Nursing. (2006b). *The healthful work environment tool kit©*. Retrieved from http://www.nln.org/docs/default-source/professional-development-programs/healthful-work-environment-toolkit.pdf?sfvrsn=2

National League for Nursing. (2017). *Leadership Institute*. Retrieved from: http://www.nln.org/professional-development-programs/leadership-programs

Nursing Organizations Alliance. (2004). *Principles and elements of a healthful practice work environment*. Lexington, KY: Author.

O'Connor, S., & Carlson, E. (2016). Safety culture and senior leadership behavior. *Journal of Nursing Administration, 46*(4), 215–220. doi:10.1097/NNA.0000000000000330

Outcalt, C. L., Faris, S. K., McMahon, K. N., & Astin, A. W. (2001). *Developing non-hierarchical leadership on campus: Case studies and best practices in higher education*. Westport, CT: Greenwood Publishing Group.

Patterson, B. J., & Krouse, A. M. (2015). Competencies for leaders in nursing education. *Nursing Education Perspectives*, *36*(2), 76–82. doi:10.5480/13-1300

Pennsylvania Action Coalition. (2017). *Leadership*. Retrieved from http://paactioncoalition.org/index.php/initiatives/leadership

Regan, S., Wong, C., Laschinger, H. K., Cummings, G., Leiter, M., MacPhee, M., ... Read, R. (2017). Starting out: Qualitative perspectives of new graduate nurses and nurse leaders on transition to practice. *Journal of Nursing Management*, *25*, 246–255. doi:10.1111/jonm.12456

Siddique, M. A., Aslam, H. D., Khan, M., & Fatima, U. (2011). Impact of academic leadership on faculty's motivation, and organization effectiveness in higher education system. *International Journal of Business and Social Sciences*, *2*(8), 184–191.

Specht, J. A. (2013). Mentoring relationships and the levels of role conflict and role ambiguity experienced by novice nursing faculty. *Journal of Professional Nursing*, *29*(5), e25-e31. doi:10.1016/j.profnurs.2013.06.006

Steege, L. M., Pinekenstein, B. J., Arsenault Knudsen, É., & Rainbow, J. G. (2017). Exploring nurse leader fatigue: A mixed methods study. *Journal of Nursing Management*, *25*(4), 276–286. doi:10.1111/jonm.12464

Wagner, J. I. J., Cummings, G., Smith, D. L., Olson, J., Anderson, L., & Warren, S.

(2010). The relationship between structural empowerment and psychological empowerment for nurses: A systematic review. *Journal of Nursing Management*, *18*, 448–462. doi:10.1111/j.1365-2834.2010.01088.x

Wolf, G., Triolo, P., & Ponte, P. (2008). Magnet Recognition Program: The next generation. *Journal of Nursing Administration*, *38*(4), 200–204. doi:10.1097/01.NNA.0000312759.14536.a9

Wong, C. A., Laschinger, H. K., MacDonald-Rencz, S., Burkoski, V., Cummings, G., D'Amour, D. ... Grau, A. (2013). Part 2: Nurses' career aspirations to managerial roles: Qualitative findings from a national study of Canadian nurses. *Journal of Nursing Management*, *21*, 231–241. doi:10.1111/j.1365-2834.2012.01451.x

Young, P. K., Pearsall, C., Stiles, K. A., Nelson, K., & Horton-Deutsch, S. (2011). Becoming a nursing faculty leader. *Nursing Education Perspectives*, *32*(4), 222–228. doi:10.5480/1536-5026-32.4.222

Zwarenstein, M., Goldman, J., & Reeves, S. (2009). Interprofessional collaboration: Effects of practice-based interventions on professional practice and health care outcomes. *Cochrane Database of Systematic Reviews*, *8*(3). doi:10.1002/14651858.CD000072.pub2

8

Competency VI: Pursue Continuous Quality Improvement in the Nurse Educator Role

Theresa M. "Terry" Valiga, EdD, RN, CNE, ANEF, FAAN

Today's health care environment is characterized by uncertainty, ambiguity, constant technological advances, knowledge explosion, calls for interprofessional practice and collaborative learning, calls for evidence-based practices in all arenas, and, among other things, constant change. In fact, the rate of change in all areas of our lives and professional practice makes it impossible for all but the most scholarly futurists to envision what tomorrow's environment will be like.

Within this context, nursing education must remain current and relevant, and it is the work of nurse educators to ensure that goal is reached. Nurse educators themselves, therefore, must remain current regarding societal, educational, technological, health care, and nursing practice changes. They also must know and use relevant pedagogical evidence to design curricula that will prepare graduates to thrive in—and help shape— an unknown and uncertain future, to employ innovative strategies that fully engage learners in the learning process, to "live" a student-centered philosophy, and to use appropriate methods to assess and evaluate students' knowledge, skills, and professional identity formation.

Competency VI: Pursue Continuous Quality Improvement in the Nurse Educator Role and its accompanying list of descriptive behaviors outlined by the National League for Nursing (NLN, 2012) remains a crucial area for all educators but perhaps most especially for those who work to prepare nurses who will provide care, teach, influence public policy, enhance systemwide performance, and conduct research. A review of research in nursing and other fields supports this assertion as noted in the narrative that follows.

Nurse educators recognize that their role is multidimensional and that an ongoing commitment to develop and maintain competence in the role is essential. To effectively pursue continuous quality improvement in the educator role, the nurse educator

> demonstrates a commitment to lifelong learning;

> recognizes that career enhancement needs and activities change as experience is gained in the role;

> participates in professional development opportunities that increase one's effectiveness in the educator role;

> balances the teaching, scholarship, and service demands inherent in the role of educator and member of an academic institution;

> uses feedback gained from self, peer, student, and administrative evaluation to improve one's effectiveness in the educator role;

> engages in activities that promote socialization to the educator role;

> uses knowledge of legal and ethical issues relevant to higher education and nursing education as a basis for influencing, designing, and implementing policies and procedures related to students, faculty, and the educational environment; and

> mentors and supports faculty colleagues.

REVIEW OF THE LITERATURE

The Cumulative Index to Nursing and Allied Health Literature (CINAHL), PubMed, and Education Resources Information Center (ERIC) were searched for articles published in English between 2005 and 2017 using the following search terms that reflect concepts evident in the previously listed competency and/or task statements: lifelong learning, socialization to the educator role, professional development, mentoring, networking, use of feedback, and workload balance. Such broad terms yielded 9,800 articles. Excluding nonresearch articles, articles that address the faculty role outside the United States or Canada, and articles specific to faculty in the liberal arts resulted in a total of 296 titles that seemed relevant. The abstracts of these 296 articles were reviewed, and the 87 that address concepts related to career development stages were read in full. The literature included in this summary, therefore, reflects selections from these 87 articles and addresses initial socialization to the educator role, developing confidence and expertise in the role, functioning as a leader in the role, and facing the challenges inherent in the role. For each stage of development, strategies for continuous quality improvement are noted, all in an effort to help the nurse educator fully meet Competency VI by demonstrating the behaviors outlined.

Initial Socialization to the Role

While primary and secondary education teachers are required to be prepared as teachers, educators who teach in colleges and universities typically have no such requirements for appointment to a faculty position. The prevailing assumption is that if one knows one's field—English literature, philosophy, biology, nursing practice, and so forth—one can effectively help others learn that field. The result of this paradigm is that many college and university nurse faculty come into the role with little or no understanding of the academic culture (other than what they may have gained from being students themselves), expectations of the role, best ways to facilitate learning, complexities of the role, or ways to meet the professional identity formation needs of increasingly diverse student populations. They are given teaching assignments and expected to implement the role at the same level of expertise they demonstrated as clinicians.

In a study of accredited prelicensure nursing program administrators, however, Poindexter (2013) found that the expectations regarding novice nurse educators' knowledge and skill were quite high, despite the fact that many such individuals have no formal preparation in teaching. Survey respondents in this study (*n* = 450–479, depending on the question) were asked to identify the minimal expected proficiency level—based on Benner's "novice-to-expert" categories (1984)—of each nurse educator competency (noted by the NLN and/or in the literature) for an entry-level novice nurse educator to assume a full-time, non–tenure- and tenure-track teaching position within their institution. Poindexter found that more than 50 percent of respondents expected novice faculty to be at least *competent* in all areas and 20 percent to 30 percent expected them to be *proficient* in most areas; few expected novice faculty to be *expert* in most areas. She noted that expectations related to competencies differed among types of institutions (i.e., community college, liberal arts colleges, research-intensive universities) and the position into which an individual was being hired (i.e., tenure or nontenure track), but despite these differences, she concluded that "the need for educators to assume positions within academic environments in the numbers that are projected across the United States will require careful planning to prepare nurses with the competencies and skills needed to successfully transition into their academic roles" (p. 565).

One of the competencies included in Poindexter's (2013) study was that of *nursing practice*, meaning that nurse educators are expected to maintain their clinical competence/expertise, as well as develop and maintain competence as educators. The model of clinician-educators is prevalent in schools of medicine, and gaining a deeper understanding of this role and its expectations was the focus of a mixed-methods study completed in Canada by Sherbino, Frank, and Snell (2014). Through focus groups with 22 deans of medicine and directors of medical education centers, as well as a survey of 350 deans, academic chairs, and residency program directors, these researchers found that 85 percent of respondents agreed or strongly agreed that physicians with advanced training in medical education are needed to serve as clinician-educators. The researchers concluded by defining a clinician-educator as "a clinician active in health professional practice who applies theory to education practice, engages in education scholarship, and serves as a consultant to other health professionals on education issues" (p. 1). Although there was no clear endorsement for any particular type of training for clinician-educators, 55 percent of survey respondents agreed or strongly agreed that a master's degree in education is effective preparation, and 39 percent agreed or strongly agreed that faculty development programs are effective. Thus, while this study was conducted in Canada and in relation to medical educators, it informs our understanding of the socialization of novice nurse educators, suggesting that (1) such socialization must attend to helping them develop a broad range of abilities, while maintaining their clinical skills, and (2) some type of "formal" preparation for the educator role is important.

In an attempt to understand the experience of novice nurse educators as they transition into an academic role, Cooley and De Gagne (2016) undertook a hermeneutic phenomenological qualitative study using audio recordings and verbatim transcripts of interviews, along with journal data describing day-to-day experiences in the role. The study was designed to gain insight about novice nurse faculty's experience in academia, to examine their perceptions of facilitators and barriers to the development of nurse educator practice competence, and to identify transformative learning experiences related to novice faculty development. Participants were master's-prepared nurse clinicians who had taught theory and clinical components to prelicensure nursing students for less than three academic years. Seven faculty teaching in a private, religious-based, four-year college participated in the study.

Participants in the Cooley and De Gagne (2016) study characterized the socialization experience as having a wide range of challenges and as "exciting yet terrifying" and "a little overwhelming but intriguing," and they identified barriers and facilitators to their transition into academia. Barriers included the following: insufficient time to do all that was expected of them, discrepancies regarding what those expectations were, insufficient knowledge regarding teaching/learning and the faculty role, lack of confidence, and lack of a mentorship program. Their transition was facilitated by the following: formal education regarding the faculty role, the advice/guidance/support provided by others, feedback from student evaluations, and their own commitment to student learning and excellence in all they do. The findings from this study suggest that novice nurse educators may need to be more deliberate in the interview and hiring process to inquire about the developmental support that will be available to them when they join the faculty to ensure the guidance they receive will be less sporadic, limited, and lacking in precision for the specific situations they will confront as new faculty, as was reported by participants in this study. They may also need to seek out an extended mentorship relationship with "a devoted mentor to guide and direct the on-the-job learning," which Cooley and De Gagne (2016, p. 99) found to be an essential factor in developing the new nurse educator's competence. They noted that the experiences of new faculty in the unfamiliar academic setting are likely novel and often unexpected, and they require a wealth of new knowledge and time, support, and guidance from others to be successful in the role.

In summary, the literature increasingly documents the need for new faculty to have a sound knowledge base regarding teaching principles, student/teacher relationships, curriculum design, and assessment of learning and academic policies, in addition to maintaining their practice expertise. The studies reported here also document the need for new faculty to receive academic or "on the job" preparation for the complex role they are about to undertake, as well as a strong support system—including a mentor—to enhance their success. Individuals transitioning into a nurse educator role would be wise, therefore, to inquire about such expectations, resources, and support, and to collaborate with their dean, director, mentor, or other person at the school to formulate a clear plan to prepare fully for the multidimensional faculty role.

Developing Confidence and Expertise in the Role

As nurse educators move beyond the initial socialization stage, new demands are placed on them, and additional contributions are expected of them. Faculty who are at midcareer need different support systems and resources to keep their teaching vibrant and current, strengthen their scholarly contributions, advance in rank, and assume new responsibilities within a school of nursing.

Bittner and O'Connor (2012) conducted a descriptive, quantitative study in the New England region to determine barriers to job satisfaction as reported by nurse faculty. Deans/directors of all NLN member schools (diploma, associate degree, baccalaureate/

higher degree) in Connecticut, Maine, Massachusetts, New Hampshire, Rhode Island, and Vermont were asked to invite all their full-time and part-time faculty to participate in the study by responding to a survey. Based on responses from 226 nurse faculty to the 32-item survey, which asked about workload, satisfaction, and identified barriers to satisfaction, these researchers found that a healthful work environment and manageable workload were essential to job satisfaction. Thus, even as nurse educators become accustomed to the academic environment and their role in it, they need to continue to learn how to manage their workload and function in a challenging environment.

Through a cross-sectional, nonexperimental study of the professional work life of nursing faculty, Candela, Gutierrez, and Keating (2013) used a 45-item online survey to gather information about several aspects of the nurse faculty work life, including teaching competence, productivity, and organizational support. For the 808 participants—all of whom were employed in diploma, associate degree, or baccalaureate/higher degree programs accredited by the Commission on Collegiate Nursing Education (CCNE) or the Accreditation Commission for Education in Nursing (NLNAC)—the aspects of work life that significantly predicted nurse faculty members' intent to stay or leave the faculty role included the following: administration's support for faculty improvement, perceived teaching expertise, and perceptions of their own productivity (which could refer to research or other scholarly work, teaching innovations, mentoring activities, contributions to professional associations, etc.). Regarding continued growth in the educator role, this study suggested that faculty—once they have moved beyond the initial socialization phase—may need to focus their efforts on learning how to work effectively with administration, develop and pursue a plan for scholarly work and significant professional involvement/contributions, and continue to enhance their expertise as educators.

One way to enhance one's scholarly productivity was suggested by Brykczynski (2012), who used a narrative pedagogical approach that combined conventional pedagogy with action research to revise a family and health promotion course for graduate family nurse practitioner students and disseminate the outcomes of her work. This effort illustrates how nurse educators can incorporate research, evaluation, and reflection into their daily teaching practice; enhance their own scholarly productivity; and advance the scholarship of teaching. Another creative approach was described by Eddy (2007), who addressed how evaluation data that result from teaching, service, practice, and/or curriculum efforts can be used as scholarship. Both of these researchers acknowledge that, regardless of the type of academic institution in which one is employed, teachers should be expected to engage in ongoing analysis and synthesis of data to evaluate and continually improve their courses, teaching skills, learner outcomes, and overall curriculum, all of which are examples of the scholarship of teaching and constitute integral components of the practice of teaching. Thus, midcareer faculty need to learn creative ways to do all that is expected of them, including scholarly work that, for some, may focus on the scholarship of teaching.

One additional study of midcareer faculty reinforced the notion that challenges in the role continue, as do opportunities and the need for continued growth and improvement. Through interviews with an unspecified number of faculty in theology and religion who participated in a workshop on teaching for midcareer faculty, Baker-Fletcher, Carr, Menn, and Ramsay (2005) concluded that midcareer is an opportunity for deeper investment in one's teaching, learning how to successfully manage the challenges associated with competing claims for one's time, accepting the shifts in one's scholarly focus that may occur as one's interests broaden or evolve, becoming more effective in facing the challenges of an increasing generational gap between oneself and one's students, and accepting the responsibilities associated with being a longer term, more "senior" member of a faculty. It is clear that continuous quality improvement in the educator role is as important for midcareer faculty as it is for new faculty, albeit with a different focus, and that the need for continued learning and growth continues as one joins the "senior ranks" of the educational community.

Functioning as a Leader in the Role

As nurse educators advance in their careers, they are expected to provide leadership within their schools and universities, their scholarly arenas, and their professional communities. Such demands are met most effectively when educators take deliberate action to grow as leaders and change agents and continue to pursue quality in such roles. This is not to suggest that all educators need to take on administrative or management positions, since leadership and management are two related but different phenomena (Grossman & Valiga, 2017), but it is expected that our senior educators function as leaders.

The literature is replete with calls for leaders in all fields, and nursing education is no exception. Leaders are needed who have a vision of a preferred future for nursing education, articulate that vision clearly and powerfully, entice others to collaborate to achieve the vision, lead change processes that fully engage followers to achieve the vision—thereby shaping a preferred future for nursing education—and evaluate the impact of such changes (Grossman & Valiga, 2017). Leaders assume roles as guides, "cheerleaders," sources of support, spokespeople for the group, mentors, change agents, and risk takers. Educators who are seasoned in the educator role need to take on each of these leadership roles and may need to develop the leadership knowledge, skills, and values to effectively take on such challenges.

As mentioned, a key role often played by more senior faculty is that of mentor, a role that can extend even beyond retirement and that can have powerful outcomes. Heinrich and Oberleitner (2012), for example, reported on a project where what they called "scholar-mentors" engaged peers in making scholarship a cooperative venture and a collective responsibility. The outcomes of this project were increased scholarly productivity and a more positive work environment that served to attract and retain highly qualified faculty.

For her dissertation, Becker (2013) conducted a hermeneutic phenomenological study of the career trajectories of 13 "master nursing academics," as she called the participants, who could describe the phenomenon of professional identity in such faculty. All interviewees held doctoral degrees (PhD, EdD, DNP); were employed as nursing faculty members in a college offering bachelor's and master's degrees in nursing; had more than five years of academic experience; demonstrated expertise in the scholarship areas of discovery, teaching, practice, or integration; and met the criteria for a master academic, which were grounded in the American Association of Colleges of Nursing (1999) definitions of scholarship in nursing. Through a qualitative analysis of written narratives describing a defining moment in their careers, an illustrated career trajectory visual created by each participant, and narrative interviews, Baker identified the essence of professional identity in master nursing academics as being composed of the following themes: professional identity is an individualized construct, the workplace is a formative agent regarding one's professional identity, teachers are lifelong students, relationships are key in one's formation, maintaining a focus on students is critical, and one engages in constant reconstruction over time. Based on her conclusion that professional identity formation and development are a relevant phenomenon for nurse faculty throughout an entire career, one can see the need for continuous learning, self-reflection, and honest assessment of one's strengths and areas in need of improvement as one evolves and serves as a leader in the field.

Facing the Challenges Inherent in the Role

Throughout their careers, nurse educators face many challenges that may inhibit their efforts to pursue continuous quality improvement in the role. In addition to the challenge of workload mentioned previously, educators are challenged by societal changes, institutional expectations, and shifting self-confidence, all of which can lead to role strain. As one implements the nurse educator role, one is presented with many reasons to pursue continuous quality improvement to remain effective in the role and ensure that our curricula, learning goals, strategies to facilitate student learning, and methods to assess learning and evaluate performance remain relevant, particularly in light of the changing dynamics in nursing, health care, and education.

Messinger (2011), for example, highlighted the challenges of working with students and faculty who are increasingly diverse. Using oral history interviews with 30 faculty members working to secure lesbian, gay, bisexual, and transgender (LGBT)-supportive policies on their respective campuses, this researcher identified reasons the faculty members became involved in this advocacy, types of advocacy in which they engaged, factors associated with engaging in advocacy, and challenges facing these faculty advocates.

Increasingly, faculty are challenged to consider legal aspects of their role, whether the concerns center on accommodations for students with disabilities, documenting a failing grade in a course or in clinical performance, or disciplining students. Thus, having a grasp of legal knowledge can be particularly helpful to those who educate future professionals. Meyer (2007), for example, reviewed representative court decisions that involved disciplining students and noted that doing so for reasons other than purely academic concerns can lead to legal challenges. He concluded that even the most balanced, ethical, and informed approach to student discipline cannot prevent all lawsuits, but being aware of one's legal responsibilities can better position an educator should such challenges occur.

Certainly, issues of academic integrity are of concern to nurse educators, whether they teach in face-to-face or online environments. Morgan and Hart (2013) conducted a quasi-experimental study to investigate an academic integrity (AI) intervention in an online RN-to-BSN nursing program. Students newly admitted to this program were randomly assigned to a control group ($n = 169$), which received the usual honor code exposure, or a treatment group ($n = 177$), which received a faculty-designed intervention. Responses to a survey tool completed at the end of the semester revealed that self-reported cheating was very low in both groups; students in the treatment group, however, reported higher levels of faculty and student support for AI policies and perceived these policies to be more effective ($p < .05$). They concluded that while more research is needed in the area of AI, especially in postlicensure nursing students, faculty-initiated discussions appear to foster a culture of AI. Faculty would do well, therefore, to continue to develop their understanding of the concept of academic integrity and ways to promote it in their schools of nursing.

One particular academic integrity issue faced by many educators is that of cheating. In an effort to identify policies and practices that deter cheating in nursing education, Stonecypher and Willson (2014) conducted a systematic literature review to assess the evidence available related to this challenge. Their review of 43 articles that met their inclusion criteria revealed that clearly defined behaviors, processes, and consequences are essential to guide implementation of specific cheating deterrent strategies. Since it is faculty who develop and approve such policies and processes, it is essential that educators learn about why students cheat, how student-teacher relationships can promote or deter cheating, legal considerations when addressing claims of cheating, and other elements of the phenomenon.

A final challenge to be addressed is that of incivility. Early work by Clark and Springer (2007) used an interpretive qualitative method to examine student and faculty perceptions of incivility in nursing education, possible causes of incivility, and potential remedies. Fifteen of 36 faculty and 168 of 467 students in the associate and baccalaureate degree nursing programs of a metropolitan public university completed the Incivility in Nursing Education survey, which included four open-ended questions. The findings led these researchers to conclude that both nurse faculty and students perceive incivility as a problem both in and out of the classroom, and such incivility often stems from stress, disrespect, faculty arrogance, and a sense of student entitlement. Clark, Olender, Kenski, and Cardoni (2013) extended this and other work on incivility and provided evidence that faculty-to-faculty incivility is "alive and well" in nursing education. Additionally, Suplee, Lachman, Siebert, and Anselmi (2008) noted that the growing trend in uncivil behavior has led faculty to be guarded in their interactions with students, which often leads to what can be perceived as unwillingness of faculty to reach out to students. These researchers cited numerous case studies and offered practical and legal analyses of incivility in the classroom, clinical setting, and online environment; they concluded by suggesting the critical need for faculty development and policy generation.

The challenges noted here are but a few of those nurse faculty face. The realities of increased integration of technology into our everyday lives and education; widening generation gaps between students and faculty; heightened demands for "covering it all" while, at the same time, knowledge is exploding at an unprecedented rate; greater expectations regarding program outcomes (e.g., licensing and certification exam pass rates); and continued expectations of employers that graduates are fully prepared to enter the job market and "hit the ground running"—along with other social, economic, legal, political, educational, and general societal trends—will only expand the challenges faculty face as they implement their multifaceted role. It is critical, therefore, that all nurse educators engage in a variety of activities to ensure continuous quality improvement in the role, regardless of where they are along their career trajectory—novice, midcareer, or senior.

IDENTIFIED GAPS IN THE LITERATURE

While the summary provided here is by no means complete regarding the research that has been completed regarding the continuous quality improvement in the nurse educator role, several gaps are evident regarding what we know and understand about this phenomenon and what we are yet to fully grasp. One clear gap relates to the ongoing failure of higher education in general—and nursing education in particular—to insist on preparation for the teaching/educator role. Despite findings that reveal the limited understanding of the full scope of the faculty role, schools continue to appoint individuals to faculty positions who have no preparation for the role, nor do they require new faculty to engage in activities that will enhance the transition from expert clinician to novice educator.

Additionally, there is limited information about the ongoing learning needs of midcareer or senior faculty. The implication of this is that once faculty are "on board" and "figure out" what their role is, they do not have unique needs related to continued development in the role except, perhaps, the need to continually enhance their research and grant-writing skills, along with the ability to form and lead interprofessional research teams. There is little attention paid to how schools can help midcareer faculty be effective course leaders, curriculum committee chairs, or pedagogical scholars. And there is limited discussion of how senior faculty can be helped to effectively mentor their junior colleagues, challenge the status quo, and exert leadership within their communities without necessarily taking on an administrative role.

Finally, several of the gaps identified in the first edition of this book (Halstead, 2007) remain, though they have not been cited specifically in this narrative. A more comprehensive understanding is needed regarding the factors that contribute to satisfaction in the role; ways to identify and meet the role development needs of part-time and clinical-only faculty; new approaches to determining a reasonable workload and managing it successfully; and the most effective ways to evaluate faculty and identify "master teachers" or "master nursing academics," as Becker (2013) called them.

PRIORITIES FOR FUTURE RESEARCH

There would seem to be no question that Competency VI—Continuous Quality Improvement in the Nurse Educator Role—is essential if nurse educators are to continue to design and implement effective learning experiences for students, grow as professionals, and provide the leadership that is needed to shape a preferred future for nursing education and the profession as a whole. They must demonstrate a commitment to lifelong learning; recognize that career enhancement is needed even as experience is gained in the role; be able to successfully balance the multiple dimensions of this complex role; and use feedback from self, peer, student, and administrative evaluations to improve their effectiveness in the role.

In light of the need to pursue continuous quality improvement in the nurse educator role (Competency VI) so that faculty can meet the behaviors that define this goal, the nursing education community would benefit from answers to the following research questions:

> What are the most effective and efficient ways to prepare novice faculty for the complexities of the educator role and ensure a smoother transition in the role?

> What models are most effective in supporting the ongoing development of "clinician-educators" (Sherbino et al., 2014) who maintain an active clinical practice while implementing the full scope of the faculty role?

> How are the needs of novice, midcareer, and senior nursing faculty similar or different as perceived by faculty and administrators?

> What is the impact on student learning and engagement when their learning is guided by "master teachers"?

> What strategies are most effective in helping midcareer faculty make a deeper investment in their teaching, learn how to successfully manage the challenges associated with competing claims for their time, accept the shifts in their scholarly focus that may occur as their interests broaden or evolve, become more effective in facing the challenges of an increasingly diverse student population, and accept the responsibilities associated with being a longer term, more "senior" member of a faculty (all of which were identified by Baker-Fletcher et al., 2005)?

> What strategies are most effective in helping senior faculty be effective mentors to their junior colleagues and provide leadership within their schools and the education community to ensure that academic programs are relevant, evidence based, and "cutting edge"?

References

American Association of Colleges of Nursing. (1999). *Defining scholarship for the discipline of nursing*. Retrieved from http://www.aacnnursing.org/News-Information/Position-Statements-White-Papers/Defining-Scholarship

Baker-Fletcher, K., Carr, D., Menn, E., & Ramsay, M. J. (2005). Taking stock at mid-career: Challenges and opportunities for faculty. *Teaching Theology & Religion, 8*(1), 3–10.

Becker, B. A. (2013). *The lived experience of professional identity in master nursing academics* (Doctoral dissertation, University of Minnesota).

Benner, P. (1984). *From novice to expert: Excellence and power in clinical practice*. Menlo Park, CA: Addison-Wesley.

Bittner, N. P., & O'Connor, M. (2012). Focus on retention: Identifying barriers to nurse faculty satisfaction. *Nursing Education Perspectives, 33*(4), 251–254.

Brykczynski, K. A. (2012). Teachers as researchers: A narrative pedagogical approach to transforming a graduate family and health promotion course. *Nursing Education Perspectives, 33*(4), 224–228.

Candela, L., Gutierrez, A., & Keating, S. (2013). A national survey examining the professional work life of today's nursing faculty. *Nurse Education Today, 33*(8), 853–859.

Clark, C. M., Olender, L., Kenski, D., & Cardoni, C. (2013). Exploring and addressing faculty-to-faculty incivility: A national perspective and literature review. *Journal of Nursing Education, 52*(4), 211–218.

Clark, C. M., & Springer, P. J. (2007). Thoughts on incivility: Student and faculty perceptions of uncivil behavior in nursing education. *Nursing Education Perspectives, 28*(2), 93–97.

Cooley, S. S., & De Gagne, J. C. (2016). Transformative experience: Developing competence in novice nursing faculty (Research Brief). *Journal of Nursing Education, 55*(2), 96–100.

Eddy, L. L. (2007). Evaluation research as academic scholarship. *Nursing Education Perspectives, 28*(2), 77–81.

Grossman, S., & Valiga, T. M. (2017). *The new leadership challenge: Creating the future of nursing* (5th ed.). Philadelphia, PA: F.A. Davis.

Halstead, J. A. (Ed.). (2007). *Nurse educator competencies: Creating an evidence-based practice for nurse educators*. New York, NY: National League for Nursing.

Heinrich, K. T., & Oberleitner, M. G. (2012). How a faculty group's peer mentoring of each other's scholarship can enhance retention and recruitment. *Journal of Professional Nursing, 28*(1), 5–12.

Messinger, L. (2011). A qualitative analysis of faculty advocacy on LGBT issues on campus. *Journal of Homosexuality, 58*(9), 1281–1305.

Meyer, K. E. (2007). How the courts influence teaching and student discipline: Lessons learned from case law. *Journal of Physician Assistant Education, 18*(4), 44–47.

Morgan, L., & Hart, L. (2013). Promoting academic integrity in an online RN-BSN program. *Nursing Education Perspectives, 34*(4), 240–243.

National League for Nursing. (2012). *The scope of practice for academic nurse educators (2012 revision)*. New York, NY: Author.

Poindexter, K. (2013). Novice nurse educator entry-level competency to teach: A national study. *Journal of Nursing Education, 52*(10), 559–566.

Sherbino, J., Frank, J. R., & Snell, L. (2014). Defining the key roles and competencies of the clinician-educator of the 21st century: A national mixed-methods study. *Academic Medicine, 89*(5), 1–7.

Stonecypher, K., & Willson, P. (2014). Academic policies and practices to deter cheating in nursing education. *Nursing Education Perspectives, 35*(3), 167–179.

Suplee, P. D., Lachman, V. D., Siebert, B., & Anselmi, K. K. (2008). Managing nursing student incivility in the classroom, clinical setting, and on-line. *Journal of Nursing Law, 12*(2), 68–77.

9

Competency VII: Engage in Scholarship

Barbara J. Patterson, PhD, RN, ANEF
Kristen McLaughlin, MSN, RN, CPNP-PC

Engaging in scholarship is the responsibility of all academic nurse educators as disciplinary stewards to prepare the future nursing workforce and promote optimal health care outcomes locally, nationally, and globally. Most significantly, "it is through the scholarly work of nurse educators that we expand our knowledge about student learning and identify best practices for promoting their learning and development" (Oermann, 2014, p. 370). Nurse educators acknowledge that scholarship is an integral component of the faculty role, and that teaching itself is a scholarly activity.

The evidence base for engaging in scholarship is limited; however, there is significant discussion of the topic, along with exemplars, in the literature. While Boyer's (1990) scholarship of teaching remains prominent and relevant in the discussion literature and has influenced academic nursing significantly, the empirical literature with a focus on scholarship has shifted in the past decade to specific outputs of scholarship, or scholarly productivity, and influencing factors such as strategies to enhance scholarship and the challenges involved. There is less attention in the literature to linking characteristics of a scholar and the outcomes of scholarship, specifically the impact of the translation of research outputs into evidence-based strategies and student learning to advance the science of nursing education.

Although the empirical literature seems to have shifted to scholarly outputs in the past decade, the competency of engaging in scholarship remains highly relevant in that all nurse educators need to approach their teaching practice with a spirit of inquiry. Throughout one's professional career, academic nurse educators need to balance their role in engagement in scholarship. One's degree of engagement and type of scholarship will depend on context. In some academic settings, the emphasis will be on the scholarship of teaching or the scholarship of discovery. Other academic settings will call for an integration of all of Boyer's domains (1990). Nursing education environments need to support cultures that include and respect all forms of scholarship.

To implement the role of academic nurse educator and engage effectively in scholarship, the academic nurse educator

- draws on extant literature to design evidence-based teaching and evaluation practices;
- exhibits a spirit of inquiry about teaching and learning, student development, evaluation methods, and other aspects of the role;

135

> designs and implements scholarly activities in an established area of expertise;

> disseminates nursing and teaching knowledge to a variety of audiences through various means;

> demonstrates skill in proposal writing for initiatives that include, but are not limited to, research, resource acquisition, program development, and policy development; and

> demonstrates qualities of a scholar: integrity, courage, perseverance, vitality, and creativity.

REVIEW OF THE LITERATURE

There is a consensus in the literature that scholarship is a critical facet of the nursing profession and nursing education; without it our "educational practices cannot develop further" (Oermann, 2015, p. 317). Engaging in scholarship and being a scholar are important aspects of the role for academic nurse educators (Billings, 2009). A review of the literature from 2005 to 2017 on engaging in scholarship in the academic nurse educator role generated the following themes: scholarship as a process, qualities of a scholar, scholarship in nursing academia, challenges to scholarly productivity, and strategies to enhance scholarly productivity.

A comprehensive literature search was performed using the Cumulative Index to Nursing and Allied Health Literature (CINAHL), Education Resources Information Center (ERIC), EBSCOhost, Google Scholar, and ProQuest electronic databases. The following key search terms were used to identify sources: scholarship, scholar, faculty, education, nursing education, research, spirit of inquiry, nursing, and intellectual curiosity. Empirical, theoretical, and discussion literature from peer-reviewed sources was included. To be included in the review, literature had to focus on aspects of scholarship pertaining to nurse educators or academic faculty. Literature was excluded if it was not published in English in a peer-reviewed publication or the full text was not available. The publication years were limited to 2005 to 2017 to capture the evidence that was generated subsequent to the first edition of *Nurse Educator Competencies: Creating an Evidence-Based Practice for Nurse Educators* (Halstead, 2007).

The initial literature search yielded 113 potential records that related to the key terms and search limits; of these, 8 were chapter references and 44 were from nonnursing literature. From the 113 articles, 53 were eliminated due to lack of relevance to scholarship in academia. The remaining 60 articles were selected for final thematic review. The majority of articles were discussion articles in nursing ($n = 12$); other nursing literature included empirical evidence ($n = 10$), project design ($n = 11$), and editorials ($n = 4$). Nonnursing literature originated from the disciplines of education and health sciences and were composed of a retrospective review ($n = 1$), empirical evidence ($n = 3$), discussion ($n = 11$), and project design ($n = 1$). Also included for review were four chapters from nursing textbooks, Boyer's (1990) text, and two National League for Nursing publications.

Scholarship as a Process

Scholarship has been defined as "an inquiry process that results in outcomes" (Billings, 2009, p. 204), and the scholarship of teaching in nursing is "inquiry about learning and teaching" (Oermann, 2014, p. 370). Scholarship is portrayed as an active process that adds to the body of nursing knowledge and advances nursing science. In nursing education, scholarship is more than designing courses and teaching well or reflecting on how one teaches. The process of scholarship in nursing education can be depicted as one that starts with questioning, searching for new ideas, systematic inquiry about teaching and learning, dissemination with peer review and critique, and development of the science of nursing education (Billings, 2009; Oermann, 2014, 2015). Part of the process includes innovative, creative ideas that are shared with peers to enhance teaching practice and the science of education for students and faculty (Clark & Webster, 2012; Oermann, 2014). Oermann (2014) offers strategies to transform one's teaching into scholarship starting with reflection on practice through various methods of dissemination.

Conceptualizing scholarship beyond what scholars do or scholarship outputs, such as research, publications, or grants, has been discussed by several authors (Oermann, 2014; Rolfe, 2009). While the products of scholarship provide an output that can be critiqued and shared with others, the scholarship of teaching is more. Rolfe (2009) argues that there has been a gradual shift in nursing academics from critical and creative intellectual activities to research as the main activity that represents scholarship. This argument has support from Boyer's work and his concern about "a restricted view of scholarship" (Boyer, 1990, p. 15). Rolfe's (2009) perspective is that scholarship is "something that academics do rather than something they produce" (p. 819). He suggests that a discipline that values only empirical evidence as scholarship, or output, restricts the development and advancement of nursing.

CHARACTERISTICS OF A SCHOLAR

While multiple authors have discussed the characteristics or attributes of a scholar (Conard & Pape, 2014; Grace, Willis, Roy, & Jones, 2016; Stockhausen & Turale, 2011), there is limited empirical literature to provide evidence of what constitutes a scholar. Conard and Pape (2014) noted that nursing scholars are naturally inquisitive and seek to develop new knowledge. They discussed the components of a scholar being a problem solver, thinker, collaborative partner, change agent, and innovator, while having the virtues of tenacity, intuitiveness, honesty, integrity, and trustfulness. Not accepting the status quo and looking at one's practice differently, with curiosity about what works and what does not, have been articulated by several authors as necessary scholar attributes (Emerson & Records, 2008; Smoyak, 2011; Stockhausen & Turale, 2011). Scholars devote time and energy to science (Parse, 2005), exhibit attributes of a strong work ethic (Stockhausen & Turale, 2011), and have passion and intellectual curiosity (Fung, 2017). Described as within the nature of a scholar (Frenn, 2015), a spirit of inquiry when new ideas develop is crucial to challenge how educators practice. Scholars must "uncover and expand the known and yet-to-be known of the knowledge vision" (Parse, 2005, p. 119) as this is what is essential to knowledge development for nursing education.

Consistent with these discussions are the findings of an empirical study conducted with 13 Australian nurse professorial scholars (Stockhausen & Turale, 2011). Using in-depth interviews, the researchers identified two subthemes of scholarship, that of "becoming a scholar" and "being a scholar" (p. 91). The participants addressed the ability to think differently, look at alternative views, and critically interrogate ideas as composing what it means to be a scholar. They described the attributes of scholars as having authenticity, an inquiring mind, integrity, courage, and humility; being collegial, resilient, questioning, and open to ideas; and accepting leadership responsibility (p. 92).

In reference to nursing scholars, Grace et al. (2016) describe the preferred qualities of a scholar as "able to fluidly move up and down the ladder of abstraction from concepts to the design of empirical research...capable of asking conceptual questions and be motivated to determine and critique conceptual and theoretical linkages among research areas of inquiry" (p. 63). They contend that scholars need to have a depth of understanding and be committed to the discipline's mission as disciplinary stewards. They also argue that preparing exemplary scholars who are critical thinkers is a moral imperative for the discipline.

Scholarship in Nursing Academia

Boyer's (1990) model of scholarship has been foundational for the development of the science of nursing education. The eight nurse educator core competencies and their supporting evidence from the past decade presented in this book indicate that the scholarship of teaching and learning is growing in nursing academia and informing our teaching practices. Other evidence acknowledging the scholarship of teaching includes nursing conferences focused specifically on advancing the science of nursing education, seven schools of nursing recognized as NLN Centers of Excellence for Advancing the Science of Nursing Education since 2013 (D. Hoover, personal communication, August 10, 2017), certification for nurse educators (6,004 certified nurse educators [CNEs™] since 2005) (L. Christensen, personal communication, October 12, 2017), and journals entirely devoted to research in nursing education.

Nursing academia continues to value and reward the scholarship of discovery or original research (Grace et al., 2016; Rolfe, 2009). The empirical evidence in the past decade has focused on the outputs of scholarship and influencing factors, such as doctoral faculty research, scholarly productivity and work-life balance (Smeltzer et al., 2017), and scholarly productivity and workload (Smeltzer, Sharts-Hopko, Cantrell, Heverly, & Jenkinson, 2017). Focus group data revealed workload issues, such as the faculty shortage and institutional barriers, as having a significant impact on the ability to conduct scholarship (Smeltzer et al., 2017). Based on their findings, Smeltzer et al. (2017) expressed concern about the sustainability of current workloads and scholarly productivity.

Another focal area is the recognition of different emphases on what constitutes faculty scholarship for faculty with research doctorates and clinical doctorates and, in particular, the necessary institutional support mechanisms for DNP faculty (Smeltzer et al., 2017). O'Lynn (2015) argued for scholarship diversity, with both discovery and translational research being important for the science and practice of nursing education. He also suggested that a diversity of types of scholarship may better meet the needs of different academic environments, such as those whose primary mission is teaching and not the conduct of original research. Smeltzer et al. (2017) noted that while DNP faculty are expected to engage in scholarship, they may have fewer resources and less administrative support than PhD faculty, increasing the challenge of scholarly engagement for these faculty.

Internationally, scholarly productivity has also been the focus of the nursing academic literature. Roberts and Turnbull (2005) conducted a survey of Australian nurse academics (N = 154) to examine levels of scholarly productivity. Their findings support a minimal increase in scholarly productivity from the previous five years, with a concentration on scholarship that is less rewarded in the Australian academic system, such as oral presentations. Roberts and Turnbull argue that theoretical and teaching scholarship should be given more recognition and that academic environments need to foster scholarly activities so they can thrive.

While acknowledging Boyer's contributions, Thoun (2009) cited limitations of Boyer's framework for scholarship in nursing academia and proposed a contemporary framework for nursing to capture the varied contributions of nurse educators in their teaching practices. She argues that in current teaching practice, scholarship needs to support "the combined strength inherent in the oneness of professional practice, teaching, research, administration, and community service" (p. 555). Thoun identifies three patterns of scholarship: emergent, educational and administrative, and professional.

SCHOLARSHIP IN HIGHER EDUCATION

The discussions in the higher education literature mirror many of the same concerns that academic nurse educators have expressed, such as the need to move away from an emphasis solely on products of scholarship to incorporate more inclusive forms of scholarship. In a review of the literature in higher education and academic health sciences, it is argued that the impact of metrics (Bonnell, 2016) and the quantification of scholarship may contribute to the devaluation of teaching (Crookes, Smith, Else, & Crookes, 2016; Oravec, 2017; Stromquist, 2017), the scholarship of engagement (Smesny et al., 2007), and what constitutes scholarship and its accompanying challenges. This shift may impact the questions a discipline asks or does not ask (Manarin & Abrahamson, 2016) and thus the development of knowledge. With changing conceptions of scholarship, recognizing scholarship more broadly and encouraging academics to articulate the impact of their work are crucial (Crookes et al., 2016). Additionally, another consideration is that other forms of scholarship, such as the scholarship of application and integration, may not be easily quantifiable. Hofmeyer, Newton, and Scott (2007) strongly advocated for embracing diversity of scholarship and "to take any necessary risks involved in changing the status quo of privileging traditional scholarship, and those who generate it" (p. 6).

In an attempt to define and further empirically differentiate good teaching, scholarly teaching, and the scholarship of teaching and learning and examine the relationships among them, Vajoczki, Savage, Martin, Borin, and Kustra (2011) surveyed all undergraduate faculty at McMaster University in Canada. Good teaching was operationalized by the principles of good practice in teaching, such as prompt feedback, time on task, faculty-student contact, and respect for diverse learning. Scholarly teaching was defined as including reflection on teaching, using evidence-informed approaches, attending conferences, collegial discussions, and engagement in the literature. The key distinction with the scholarship of teaching and learning was the inclusion of dissemination of scholarship beyond the local context with external critique. Findings from the survey (N = 339, 14 percent response rate) support a strong correlation among good teaching and scholarly teaching and the scholarship of teaching and learning. The perceived value of teaching varied across faculties, with the faculty of health sciences more strongly agreeing that teaching was valued.

The scholarship of engagement (Boyer, 1996) has received significantly more attention in the higher education literature (Franz, 2016; Giles, 2008; Kasworm & Abdrahim, 2014; Sandmann, Saltmarsh, & O'Meara, 2008) than in the nursing literature. In 1996, Boyer argued that "the academy must become a more vigorous partner in the search for answers to our most pressing social, civic, economic, and moral problems" (p. 11). Engaged scholarship calls for a greater emphasis on impact to solve society's wicked problems (Fitzgerald, Bruns, Sonka, Furco, & Swanson, 2012), to engage practitioner voices (Giles, 2008), to have a broader range of scholarship (Franz, 2016), and to make an impact for good in the world (Fung, 2017). Fitzgerald et al. (2012) argued that "not all knowledge and expertise reside in the academy, and that both expertise and great learning opportunities in teaching and scholarship also reside in non-academic settings" (p. 227).

Challenges to Scholarly Productivity

The literature has been satiated in empirical evidence identifying challenges to academic nurse educators' productivity specific to Boyer's (1990) scholarship of discovery. Discussions mainly focus on the challenges of dissemination of knowledge and original research through publications in peer-reviewed journals, rather than on the challenges of dissemination through oral presentations. Lack of time, knowledge, and/or confidence are the most prevalent themes identified by nurse educators as negatively impacting scholarly productivity (Keen, 2007; Lehna, Hermanns, Monsivais, & Engebretson, 2016; Smesny et al., 2007; Wheeler, Hardie, Schell, & Plowfield, 2008).

A descriptive, correlational study links both nurse educators aged in their 40s and educators holding higher academic ranks as perceiving a greater importance for publication, with doctoral faculty being the most likely to have the majority of scholarly output (Roberts & Turnbull, 2005). Both nationally and globally, pursuance of a doctoral degree later in nurse faculty careers is recognized as placing a limit on the number of years remaining to contribute toward scholarship (Oyama et al., 2015; Smesny et al., 2007; Wheeler et al., 2008).

The nurse faculty shortage resonates in the literature as contributing significantly to barriers to participation in scholarship. The shortage requires faculty to devote more time toward the process of teaching rather than to the scholarship of teaching and learning; also, senior faculty retirements have left a paucity of faculty-scholars to mentor novice faculty (Heinrich, Hurst, Leigh, Oberleitner, & Poirrier, 2009; Heinrich & Oberleitner, 2012; Smesny et al., 2007; Wheeler et al., 2008). Smeltzer et al. (2017) conducted a national study that evaluated doctoral faculty perceptions regarding the effects of increased doctoral enrollments on doctoral faculty scholarly productivity. Findings reveal increased doctoral faculty workloads, increased administrative responsibilities, and the shortage of nurse educators in academia as challenges affecting the time available for scholarship activity. While the sample proved to be homogenous toward the national profile of doctoral nurse educators, Smeltzer and colleagues (2017) identify a study limitation as failing "to achieve a sample reflecting the national distribution of PhD versus DNP programs" (p. 201).

Increased demands placed on faculty to devote to their teaching practices potentiate challenges with time allocation between the practice of teaching and the scholarship of teaching. The NLN-Carnegie National Survey (Kaufman, 2007, p. 297) identified that 62 percent of faculty expressed having scholarly activity time commitments outside of their primary academic institution workloads, during both the school year and break periods. Furthermore, changing academic climates toward online teaching environ-ments, larger class sizes, and the commitment of educators to stay abreast of and apply evidence-based teaching strategies to practice present additional challenges to the demands on faculty time (Smeltzer et al., 2014, 2017). A quantitative survey of Japanese nursing faculty ($N = 400$, 39.7 percent response rate) mirrored national findings that increased teaching workloads detract from scholarly productivity (Oyama et al., 2015).

In a retrospective literature review conducted from 1980 to February 2006, Smesny et al. (2007) identified the common challenges to scholarship among multidiscipline health sciences faculty. Unique to health sciences faculty was the "requirement to provide clinical services and to participate in clinical teaching activities...which limits the avail-able time for the faculty member to engage in scholarly activities" (Smesny et al., 2007, p. 4). Lack of mentorship for scholarship, lack of faculty awareness of the different types of scholarly activities, and an institutional culture not supportive of scholarship were other common barriers found among medicine, nursing, pharmacy, and dentistry faculty.

The empirical evidence proposes that deficiencies within institutional and admin-istrative support for doctoral faculty create further challenges to scholarly productiv-ity. Smeltzer et al. (2016) identified institutional and administrative resources as including "startup funding, interdisciplinary collaboration, research and teaching assistants, office of research and support, formal and informal mentoring, and...a grant writer" (p. 189). Oyama et al. (2015) indicate that difficulties in research productivity also stem from a lack of institutional support in providing research assistants. In a descriptive study evaluat-ing collaboration between DNP- and PhD-prepared faculty, qualitative findings from four focus groups revealed that overall organizational support for doctoral research and scholarship activity was deficient; this was particularly identified by DNP-prepared fac-ulty (Staffileno, Murphy, & Carlson, 2017).

In conjunction with the challenges of time and support, the concept of confidence in the educator role has evolved in the literature as another specific challenge to scholarly productivity. It was suggested that a lack of educational preparation for the educator role challenges the personal formation of identity as scholar (Heinrich & Oberleitner, 2012). Heinrich (2017) suggested the concept of scholar-imposter, as one who does not internal-ize the identity of a scholar, either from educational preparation, confidence level, or lack of a "scholar-mentor" (p. 95). This scholar-identity challenge is compounded by the trend of institutional hiring practices to fill faculty vacancies with master's-prepared and recent graduates of doctoral programs (novice scholars) and the retirement of senior faculty scholar-mentors.

Analogous to the formation of a scholar identity, the literature conveys lack of self-confidence (Houfek et al., 2010), knowledge in research skills (Oyama et al., 2015), and writ-ing skills (Keen, 2007; Wilson, Sharrad, Rasmussen, & Kernick, 2013) as personal variables that challenge nurse educator engagement in scholarship. Absence of self-confidence was recognized as having a negative impact on the ability of educators to identify issues of significance and generate questions for exploration that have a potential to expand knowledge within nursing science and nursing education (Houfek et al., 2010; Keen, 2007). The empirical evidence is focused on how challenges in self-confidence and knowl-edge affect engagement in the scholarship of discovery and the scholarship of teaching through submissions of scholarly output, rather than on how these deficiencies affect the processes of scholarship of integration and application.

Strategies to Enhance Scholarly Productivity

The majority of articles addressing strategies to enhance scholarly productivity are discussion articles that are anecdotal in nature; limited empirical evidence was found in the literature on this topic. The literature provides exemplars of projects that were designed to build scholarship capacity in programs (Cash & Tate, 2008; Chaudhry & Prelock, 2012; Jerardi et al., 2016). The themes relate to enhancing both scholarship output and outcomes through the creation of cultures and communities of scholarship, and through the provision of faculty support and the facilitating of faculty goal setting.

A primary mission of PhD programs, specific to nursing science, is to prepare nurse scholars. A culture of scholarship is inherent in these nursing programs through engagement of doctoral students in critical inquiry, philosophical discussions of assumptions and beliefs related to nursing knowledge, and mentorship of students in designing and disseminating evidence. This environment, geared toward creating cultures of scholarship within nursing education, is further recognized through the NLN Centers of Excellence in Nursing Education™ program, specifically in the category of Creating Environments That Advance the Science of Nursing Education (National League for Nursing [NLN], 2017). This program acknowledges academic nursing organizations that have established environments that advance the science of nursing education through "sustained, evidence-based, and substantive innovation; conduct ongoing research to document the effectiveness of such innovation; set high standards for themselves; and are committed to continuous quality improvement" (NLN, 2017, p. 3).

An effective strategy in enhancing scholarship is building a community of scholars (Meleis, 2012). Nurse educators in 12 Canadian Association Schools of Nursing (CASN) recognized the magnitude effect that a community of scholars had on building networks, opening dialogue, igniting spirits of inquiry, sharing innovations, and enriching scholarly activity (Cash & Tate, 2012). Oermann (2015) acknowledged that the road to scholarship in nursing education requires self-reflection, discussing ideas with colleagues, and inviting public critique. This process presents opportunity for nurse educators to reflect, evaluate, and expand current knowledge together as a community. Dissemination of knowledge is an imperative step of this process, as it enables "educational innovations" (Oermann, 2015, p. 320) to be widely shared, thereby contributing to the existing body of knowledge in nursing education.

Bosso, Hastings, Speedie, and Rodriquez de Bittner (2015) made recommendations to create "an academic environment that accommodates and nurtures scholarship" (p. 3) within pharmacy academic settings; these recommendations also have applicability to guidelines within institutions of higher education in nursing. Their recommendations include institutional leadership fostering cultures of scholarship with an impetus to generate creativity and innovation in faculty, clear delineation of institutional expectations for types of scholarship necessary for promotion and tenure, and mentorship by senior scholars. Jerardi et al. (2016) report on a national faculty development program that fosters the scholarship of teaching in pediatric medical faculty through an emphasis on the process of evaluation of "curricular innovations, evaluation tools, and teaching methodologies" (p. 4).

Institutional resources and support have been identified by several authors as critical to facilitate scholarship development. Chaudhry and Prelock (2012) presented data on an institutional initiative to enhance faculty research and scholarship endeavors by (1) providing research incentive grants to provide funding to pilot research that potentially would secure external funding, (2) supporting personnel to facilitate grant submissions, and (3) offering grant writing workshops (p. 54). Their research initiative was productive in increasing faculty scholarly activity with a noted increase in "extramural grant applications, funding, and publications" (p. 55). In the national survey conducted by Smeltzer et al. (2016), doctoral faculty reported startup funding as being the most supportive institutional resource to increase faculty scholarly productivity, with interdisciplinary collaboration on research the second most influential support for faculty. Roberts and Turnbull (2005) stated that "a workplace environment that is appropriately supported by adequate resources may be as important as the research training that can occur through mentoring" (p. 60).

Individual scholarship development has been documented to have an impact on institutions. The Robert Wood Johnson Foundation's Nurse Faculty Scholars Program was developed to promote junior faculty growth and enhance institutional research infrastructure (McBride et al., 2017). In a descriptive study, data were collected from deans/directors through open-ended telephone interviews and a survey to determine their perceptions of the impact of scholars' participation in the program and the influence on the school of nursing's research portfolio. The findings supported individual scholar growth and development as faculty members, researchers, and leaders in nursing academia. Scholars had a wider influence within their schools and universities, as well as regionally and nationally, and participation in the program contributed to schools meeting their institutional expectations "most of the time" (McBride et al., 2017, p. 6).

Wilson et al. (2013) illuminated the perceived pressures to "publish or perish" (p. 210) in nursing academics. These authors outlined an innovative institutional strategy of providing publication workshops with an overall intent to change the climate surrounding publication, from a negative shroud to that of a rewarding experience that increased "knowledge, confidence, and motivation" (p. 214). The literature further supports writing groups as an effective approach in developing communities of scholars among nurse educators, as well as a strategy to enhance faculty scholarship output (Houfek et al., 2010; Keen, 2007; Wilson et al., 2013). Teaching portfolios are recognized as a credible source of documentation of scholarship output and outcomes. These portfolios provide an opportunity for formative assessment of individual teaching, as well as a source for evaluation of individual scholarship of teaching and learning (Corry & Timmons, 2009; Oermann, 2015).

Limited discussion was found in the literature specific to the theme of goal setting for nurse educators as a means to achieve scholarship activity. Bartlett, Shattell, and Rossen (2008) introduced the concept of physically tracking scholarship, using a whiteboard, as a means to keep track of ideas and organize thoughts, and as a motivational incentive in visualizing goals and achieved scholarship activity. Another discussion relates to setting goals focused on the ability of doctoral faculty to sustain their engagement in scholarship when they set clear limits with students and with undertakings assumed within professional organizations (Smeltzer et al., 2016).

The concept of mentorship resonates as a paramount strategy for enhancing scholarship among nurse educators. The literature defines mentorship in relation to the provision of focused guidance (Bruner, Dunbar, Higgins, & Martyn, 2016), support circles (Heinrich et al., 2009; Lehna et al., 2016), and collaboration in scholarly activity through publication workshops (Wilson et al., 2013). Focus group interviews, conducted by Staffileno et al. (2017), reveal opportunities for mentorship between PhD and DNP educators by (1) matching a PhD faculty mentor with a DNP educator to facilitate dissemination of scholarship output and (2) matching a PhD educator (functioning as a DNP adviser) with a DNP faculty mentor to guide PhD faculty through the expectations of the DNP curriculum and proposals. Roberts and Turnbull (2005) found mentorship more likely to occur in support circles having both community and cultures of scholarship.

Bruner et al. (2016) surveyed nurse educators ($N = 38$, response rate 60 percent) regarding best practices for mentorship programs in nursing. The respondents included educators of all academic ranks and varied academic tracks from a single southeastern school of nursing. Formal mentorship was preferred by all educators, regardless of academic track. Priority needs identified for this school of nursing included "guidance on timely publications, mentorship on work-life balance...putting together a promotion package, guidance on test writing, and utilizing technology in the classroom" (Bruner et al., 2016, p. 327). Furthermore, the researchers evaluated the gaps between priority mentorship needs and how well they were being met by mentors. The four most prevalent gaps in mentorship correlated with meeting needs related to the practice of teaching. The fifth mentoring gap related to "developing and managing a research team" (Bruner et al., 2016, p. 328). Overall, the researchers concluded mentorship is a priority in nursing education to facilitate advancement and the retention of nurse faculty in academic careers.

Empirical research is beginning to be conducted to evaluate collaborative scholarship endeavors among DNP-prepared and PhD-prepared faculty and between DNP and PhD students (Edwards, Rayman, Diffenderfer, & Stidham, 2016; Staffileno et al., 2017). The clinical practice knowledge expertise of DNP-prepared faculty, combined with the theoretical and nursing science knowledge of PhD-prepared faculty, provides opportunity to identify current trends impacting health care outcomes, conduct research evaluating strategies to enhance student learning and knowledge, build innovative curricula, and prescribe and translate evidence-based interventions into academic practice. Staffileno et al. (2017) established that collaboration increases when faculty share interests and respect individual abilities.

In the context of PhD and DNP education, Edwards et al. (2016) recognized the potential influence of strategic approaches on fostering early collaboration and collegiality among DNP and PhD students through merged learning experiences, shared resources, and complementary projects. Heinrich (2016) proposed a prescription of "scholarly etiquette" to establish respectful, collaborative, working partnerships (p. 219). Building collaborative relationships among educators, researchers, and clinicians is reflective of the scholarship of integration and provides opportunities to "explore phenomena emanating from and influencing practice outcomes" (Meleis, 2012, p. 10).

IDENTIFIED GAPS IN THE LITERATURE

Over the past decade, there has been growth in the body of empirical literature focused on research outputs, such as publications, as well as strategies to facilitate scholarship output and the challenges involved. However, the empirical investigation of scholarship more broadly and the impact on the development of a science of nursing education is limited. Additional research that addresses the application and evaluation of scholarship to teaching practice and student outcomes continues to offer areas for exploration. The following gaps were identified:

> Investigation of the connection between all types of faculty scholarship and student learning

> Impact of educational preparation to increase the capacity of nurse scientists whose focus is the scientific and theoretical basis for nursing education

> Impact of the "scholarship of engagement" (Boyer, 1996) on student learning and community practice

> Scholarship with interprofessional teams while maintaining a nursing identity

> Instruments to measure scholarship outcomes beyond the quantification of outputs

> Systematic evaluation of strategic planning efforts to sustain scholarship with an ongoing nursing shortage, a changing profile of doctoral faculty, increased workloads, and greater numbers of nursing applicants

PRIORITIES FOR FUTURE RESEARCH

The following priorities for future research related to the competency of engaging in scholarship are recommended:

> What does being a scholar in nursing education mean to an academic nurse educator?

> How do nurse educators stimulate a spirit of inquiry in students to create a scholarly identity?

> How does the shifting proportion of nurse faculty with practice doctorates and those with research doctorates impact scholarship and the knowledge and science of nursing education?

> What is the impact of collaboration of practice and research doctorate-prepared academic nurse educators on the science of nursing education?

> How is the faculty shortage impacting the scholarship of teaching practice?

> What mission-appropriate strategies are most effective in fostering the scholarly identity of nurse educators in institutions with teaching as a primary mission?

References

Bartlett, R., Shattell, M. M., & Rossen, E. (2008). Visual tracking strategies to move scholarship forward. *Nurse Educator, 33*, 83–85. doi:10.1097/01. NNE.0000299514.16389.cb

Billings, D. (2009). Engaging in scholarship. In R. A. Wittmann-Price, & M. Godshall (Eds.), *Certified nurse educator review manual* (pp. 203–212). New York, NY: Springer Publishing Company.

Bonnell, A. (2016). Tide or tsunami? The impact of metrics on scholarly research. *Australian Universities' Review, 58*, 54–61.

Bosso, J. A., Hastings, J. K., Speedie, M. K., & Rodriquez de Bittner, M. (2015). Recommendations for the successful pursuit of scholarship by pharmacy practice faculty members. *American Journal of Pharmaceutical Education, 79*(1), 1–3. doi:10.5688/ajpe79104

Boyer, E. (1990). *Scholarship reconsidered: Priorities for the professoriate.* Princeton, NJ: Carnegie Foundation for the Advancement of Teaching.

Boyer, E. (1996). The scholarship of engagement. *Journal of Public Service & Outreach, 1*(1), 11–20.

Bruner, D. W., Dunbar, S., Higgins, M., & Martyn, K. (2016). Benchmarking and gap analysis of faculty mentorship priorities and how well they are met. *Nursing Outlook, 64,* 321–331. doi:10.1016/j.outlook.2016.02.008

Cash, P. A., & Tate, B. (2008). Creating a community of scholars: Using a community development approach to foster scholarship with nursing faculty. *International Journal of Nursing Education Scholarship, 5*(1), 1–11. doi:10.2202/1548-923X.1454

Cash, P. A., & Tate, B. (2012). Fostering scholarship capacity: The experience of nurse educators. *Canadian Journal for the Scholarship of Teaching and Learning, 3*(1), 1–19. doi:10.5206/cjsotl-rcacea.2012.1.17

Chaudhry, M. A., & Prelock, P. A. (2012). Enhancing the research and scholarship enterprise. *Nurse Educator, 37,* 54–55. doi:10.1097/NNE.0b013e3182461bcd

Clark, E., & Webster, B. (2012). Innovation and its contribution to the scholarship of learning and teaching. *Nurse Education Today, 32,* 729–731. doi:10.1016/j.nedt.2012.06.001

Conard, P., & Pape, T. (2014). Roles and responsibilities of the nursing scholar. *Pediatric Nursing, 40,* 87–90.

Corry, M., & Timmins, F. (2009). The use of teaching portfolios to promote excellence and scholarship in nursing education. *Nurse Education in Practice, 9,* 388–392. doi:10.1016/j.nepr.2008.11.005

Crookes, P., Smith, K., Else, F., & Crookes, E. (2016). Articulating performance expectations for scholarship at an Australian regional university. *Tertiary Education and Management, 22,* 82–97. doi:10.1080/13583883.2016.1151071

Edwards, J., Rayman, K., Diffenderfer, S., & Stidham, A. (2016). Strategic innovation between PhD and DNP programs: Collaboration, collegiality, and shared resources. *Nursing Outlook, 64,* 312–320. doi:10.1016/j.outlook.2016.02.007

Emerson, R., & Records, K. (2008). Today's challenge, tomorrow's excellence: The practice of evidence-based education. *Journal of Nursing Education, 47,* 359–370. doi:10.3928/01484834-20080801-04

Fitzgerald, H. E., Bruns, K., Sonka, S., Furco, A., & Swanson, L. (2012). The centrality of engagement in higher education. *Journal of Higher Education Outreach and Engagement, 16,* 7–28.

Franz, N. (2016). The legacy and future of a model for engaged scholarship: Supporting a broader range of scholarship. *Journal of Higher Education Outreach and Engagement, 20,* 217–221.

Frenn, M. (2015). Engage in scholarship of teaching. In L. Caputi (Ed.), *Certified nurse educator review book: The official NLN guide to the CNE exam* (pp. 113–124). Philadelphia, PA: Wolters Kluwer.

Fung, D. (2017). Strength-based scholarship and good education: The scholarship circle. *Innovations in Education and Teaching International, 54,* 101–110. doi:10.1080/14703297.2016.1257951

Giles, D. E. (2008). Understanding an emerging field of scholarship: Toward a research agenda for engaged, public scholarship. *Journal of Higher Education Outreach and Engagement, 12,* 97–106.

Grace, P. J., Willis, D. G., Roy, C., & Jones, D. A. (2016). Profession at the crossroads: A dialog concerning the preparation of nursing scholars and leaders. *Nursing Outlook, 64,* 61–70. doi:10.1016/j.outlook.2015.10.002

Halstead, J. A. (Ed.). (2007). *Nurse educator competencies: Creating an evidence-based practice for nurse educators.* New York, NY: National League for Nursing.

Heinrich, K. T. (2016). Toward a scholarly etiquette: How to keep your scholarly interactions prolific, respectful, and kind. *Nurse Educator, 41,* 219–221. doi:10.1097.NNE.0000000000000267

Heinrich, K. T. (2017). Imagine something different: How a group approach to scholarly faculty development can turn joy-stealing competition into scholarly productivity. *Journal of Professional Nursing, 33*, 95–101. doi:10.1016/j.profnurs.2016.08.008

Heinrich, K. T., Hurst, H., Leigh, G., Oberleitner, M. G., & Poirrier, G. P. (2009). The teacher-scholar project: How to help faculty groups develop scholarly skills. *Nursing Education Perspectives, 30*, 181–186.

Heinrich, K. T., & Oberleitner, M. G. (2012). How a faculty group's peer mentoring of each other's scholarship can enhance retention and recruitment. *Journal of Professional Nursing, 28*, 5–12. doi:10.1016/j.profnurs.2011.06.002

Hofmeyer, A., Newton, M., & Scott, C. (2007). Valuing the scholarship of integration and the scholarship of application in the academy for health sciences scholars: Recommended methods. *Health Research Policy and Systems, 5*, 1–8. doi:10.1186/1478-4505-5-5. Retrieved from http://www.health-policy-systems.com/content/5/1/5

Houfek, J. F., Kaiser, K. L., Visovsky, C., Barry, T. L., Nelson, A. E., Kaiser, M. M., & Miller, C. L. (2010). Using a writing group to promote faculty scholarship. *Nurse Educator, 35*, 41–45. doi:10.1097/NNE.0b013e3181c42133

Jerardi, K. E., Mogilner, L., Turner, T., Chandran, L., Baldwin, C., & Klein, M. (2016). Investment in faculty as educational scholars: Outcomes from the National Educational Scholars Program. *Journal of Pediatrics, 171*, 4–5. doi:10.1016/j.peds.2015.12.052

Kasworm, C. E., & Abdrahim, N. A. B. (2014). Scholarship of engagement and engagement of scholars: Through the eyes of exemplars. *Journal of Higher Education Outreach and Engagement, 18*, 121–147.

Kaufman, K. (2007). More findings from the NLN-Carnegie National Survey: How nurse educators spend their time. *Nursing Education Perspectives, 28*, 296–297.

Keen, A. (2007). Writing for publication: Pressures, barriers, and support strategies. *Nurse Education Today, 27*, 382–388. doi:10.1016/j.nedt.2006.05.019

Lehna, C., Hermanns, M., Monsivais, D. B., & Engebretson, J. (2016). From dissertation defense to dissemination: Jump start your academic career with a scholar mentor group. *Nursing Forum, 51*, 62–69. doi:10.1111/nuf.12124

Manarin, K., & Abrahamson, E. (2016). Troublesome knowledge of SoTL. *International Journal for the Scholarship of Teaching and Learning, 10*(2), Article 2. Retrieved from http://digitalcommons.georgiasouthern.edu/ij-sotl/vol10/iss2/2

McBride, A., Campbell, J., Barr, T., Duffy, J., Haozous, E., Mallow, J., . . . Theeke, L. (2017). The impact of the Nurse Faculty Scholars program on schools of nursing. *Nursing Outlook, 65*, 327–335. doi:10.1016/j.outlook.2017.01.013

Meleis, A. I. (2012). *Theoretical nursing* (5th ed.). Philadelphia, PA: Lippincott Williams & Wilkins.

National League for Nursing (NLN). (2017). *National League for Nursing Centers of Excellence in Nursing Education Program applicant handbook.* Retrieved from http://www.nln.org/docs/default-source/recognition-programs/coe_2018_coe_handbook.pdf?sfvrsn=6

Oermann, M. H. (2014). Defining and assessing the scholarship of teaching in nursing. *Journal of Professional Nursing, 30*, 370–375. doi:10.1016/j.profnurs.2014.03.001

Oermann, M. H. (2015). Becoming a scholar in nursing education. In M. H. Oermann (Ed.), *Teaching in nursing and role of the educator* (pp. 317–332). New York, NY: Springer Publishing Company.

O'Lynn, C. (2015). Endorsing the doctor of nursing practice pathway for nurse educators. *Journal of Nursing Education, 54*, 475–477. doi:10.3928/01484834-20150814-10

Oravec, J. A. (2017). The manipulation of scholarly rating and measurement systems: Constructing teaching excellence in an era of academic stardom. *Teaching in Higher Education, 22*, 423–436. doi:10.1080/13562517.2017.1301909

Oyama, Y., Fukahori, H., Miyashita, M., Narama, M., Kono, A., Atogami, F., . . . Yoshizawa, T. (2015). Cross-sectional online survey of research productivity in young Japanese nursing faculty. *Japan Journal of Nursing Science, 12*, 198–207. doi:10.1111/jjns.12060

Parse, R. (2005). Community of scholars. *Nursing Science Quarterly, 18*, 119. doi:10.1177/08943184052755862.

Roberts, K., & Turnbull, B. (2005). A millennial benchmark of nurse-academics' scholarly productivity. *Contemporary Nurse: A Journal for the Nursing Profession, 19*, 52–62. doi:10.5172/conu.19.1-2.52

Rolfe, G. (2009). Writing-up and writing-as: Rediscovering nursing scholarship. *Nurse Education Today, 29*, 816–820. doi:10.1016/j.nedt.2009.05.015

Sandmann, L., Saltmarsh, J., & O'Meara, K. A. (2008). An integrated model for advancing the scholarship of engagement: Creating academic homes for the engaged scholar. *Journal of Higher Education Outreach and Engagement, 12*, 47–64.

Smeltzer, S. C., Cantrell, M. A., Sharts-Hopko, N. C., Heverly, M. A., Jenkinson, A., & Nthenge, S. (2016). Assessment of the impact of teaching demands on research productivity among doctoral nursing program faculty. *Journal of Professional Nursing, 32*, 180–192. doi:10.1016/j.profnurs.2015.06.011

Smeltzer, S. C., Sharts-Hopko, N. C., Cantrell, M. A., Heverly, M. A., & Jenkinson, A. (2017). Nursing doctoral faculty perceptions related to the effect of increasing enrollments on productivity. *Nursing Education Perspectives, 38*, 201–202. doi:10.1097/01.NEP.0000000000000145

Smeltzer, S. C., Sharts-Hopko, N. C., Cantrell, M. A., Heverly, M. A., Wise, N., & Jenkinson, A. (2017). Perceptions of academic administrators of the effect of involvement in doctoral programs on faculty members' research and work-life balance. *Nursing Outlook. 65*, 753–760. doi:10.1016/j.outlook.2017.04.012

Smeltzer, S. C., Sharts-Hopko, N. C., Cantrell, M. A., Heverly, M. A., Wise, N., Jenkinson, A., & Nthenge, S. (2014). Nursing doctoral faculty perceptions of factors that affect their continued scholarship. *Journal*

of Professional Nursing, 30, 493–501. doi:10.1016/j.profnurs.2014.03.008

Smesny, A. L., Williams, J. S., Brazeau, G. A., Weber, R. J., Matthews, H. W., & Das, S. K. (2007). Barriers to scholarship in dentistry, medicine, nursing, and pharmacy practice faculty. *American Journal of Pharmaceutical Education, 71*(5), Article 91.

Smoyak, S. (2011). Developing a spirit of inquiry. *Journal of Psychosocial Nursing, 49*, 2–3. doi:10.3928/02793695-20110802-05

Staffileno, B. A., Murphy, M. P., & Carlson, E. (2017). Determinants for effective collaboration among DNP- and PhD-prepared faculty. *Nursing Outlook, 65*, 94–102. doi:10.1016/j.outlook.2016.08.003

Stockhausen, L., & Turale, S. (2011). An explorative study of Australian nursing scholars and contemporary scholarship. *Journal of Nursing Scholarship, 43*, 89–96. doi:10.1111/j.1547-5069.2010.01378.x

Stromquist, N. (2017). The professoriate: The challenged subject in US higher education. *Comparative Education, 53*, 132–146. doi:10.1080/03050068.2017.1254975

Thoun, D. S. (2009). Toward an appreciation of nursing scholarship: Recognizing our traditions, contributions, and presence. *Journal of Nursing Education, 48*, 552–556. doi:10.3928/01484834-20090716-01

Vajoczki, S., Savage, P., Martin, L., Borin, P., & Kustra, E. D. H. (2011). Good teachers, scholarly teachers and teachers engaged in scholarship of teaching and learning: A case study from McMaster University, Hamilton, Canada. *Canadian Journal for the Scholarship of Teaching and Learning, 2*(1), Article 2. doi:10.5206/cjsotl-rcacea.2011.1.2

Wheeler, E. C., Hardie, T., Schell, K., & Plowfield, L. (2008). Symbiosis—Undergraduate research mentoring and faculty scholarship in nursing. *Nursing Outlook, 56*, 9–15. doi:10.1016/j.outlook.2007.09.001

Wilson, A., Sharrad, S., Rasmussen, P., & Kernick, J. (2013). Publish or perish: Ensuring longevity in nurse education—Evaluation of a strategy to engage academics, students, and clinicians in publication activity. *Journal of Professional Nursing, 29*, 210–216. doi:10.1016/j.profnurs.2012.04.024

10

Competency VIII: Function Within the Educational Environment

Anne M. Krouse, PhD, MBA, RN-BC

Alecia Schneider Fox, PhD, APRN, FNP-BC

Nurse educators must be able to navigate, function, and lead within today's complex environments in higher education. Personally, the nurse educator must be prepared to take on the faculty role, encompassing teaching, scholarship, service, and engagement, as appropriate to the institution's and program's mission. Tied to the mission of the institution, the faculty role can be operationalized very differently in the various types of educational environments. Nurse educators must consider their professional goals and the alignment of those goals with the mission of the institution in which they choose to teach.

Within the institution, nurse educators must be prepared to function as leaders, influencing institutional changes that enhance student learning and engagement while creating an environment that is agile and responsive to external influences. This can be accomplished through active engagement in the institution's governance system. As the higher education and health care environments are becoming increasingly complex, nurse educators must also consistently scan those dynamic environments to remain aware of external influences and trends that can have an effect on nursing education. They must be prepared to not only respond to these influences but also become adept at discerning future trends. Nurse educators also need to be engaged in political and disciplinary discourse to advocate for issues that affect nursing and nursing education.

Engagement in networks and collaborations with partners, both internally and externally, are essential to create a shared vision for nursing and nursing education. Nurse educators should seek opportunities for personal leadership development to develop the skills and strategies required to fully embrace formal and informal leadership roles and create a shared vision for nursing education.

Nurse educators who demonstrate competence in functioning within the educational environment will understand the environment within which they practice their faculty role, demonstrate that they are "good citizens" of the academy, and recognize how external forces affect their role (National League for Nursing [NLN], 2012). The following statements (NLN, 2012) address the knowledge, skills, and attitudes that nurse educators must

149

have to be effective within the educational environment. To effectively function within the educational environment the nurse educator

> uses knowledge of history and current trends and issues in higher education as a basis for making recommendations and decisions on educational issues;

> identifies how social, economic, political, and institutional forces influence higher education in general and nursing education in particular;

> develops networks, collaborations, and partnerships to enhance nursing's influence within the academic community;

> determines his or her own professional goals within the context of academic nursing and the mission of the parent institution and nursing program;

> integrates the values of respect, collegiality, professionalism, and caring to build an organizational climate that fosters the development of students and teachers;

> incorporates the goals of the nursing program and the mission of the parent institution when proposing change or managing issues;

> assumes a leadership role in various levels of institutional governance; and

> advocates for nursing and nursing education in the political arena.

REVIEW OF THE LITERATURE

To provide an empirical discussion of what is known regarding the role of the nurse educator in the educational environment, a literature search of both nursing education and higher education as a whole was conducted using the following electronic databases: Cumulative Index of Nursing and Allied Health Literature (CINAHL), Educational Resources Information Center (ERIC), Google Scholar, and PsychINFO for published studies spanning the years 2005 through 2017. The following keywords were used: nursing education, higher education, educational environment, healthy work environment, faculty, leadership, policy, politics, role, faculty incivility, institutional mission, faculty governance, distance learning, academic-practice partnerships, and advocacy.

Although little empirical evidence was found, trends in higher education are presented to give context to the literature reviewed on nursing education. The overall themes that emerged from the review were being mission driven, strategically responding to trends in higher education, collaborating with internal and external constituents, creating a collegial environment, and leading the way.

Being Mission Driven

Every higher education institution is driven by its underlying mission. This mission forms the context for its educational programs, faculty roles, student life, and interactions with the community. Of particular concern to a faculty member is the balance between research/scholarship, teaching, service, and engagement. It is essential that nurse educators carefully consider their professional and personal goals and the alignment of those goals with the mission of the institution. A mismatch could create role dissatisfaction and accelerate attrition.

Additionally, nurse educators may struggle with integrating the clinical role with the academic faculty role. Schriner (2007) qualitatively examined the transition of nurse educators from a clinical practice role to a faculty role through an examination of the values and beliefs of seven nurses at one midwestern university who were new to the faculty role. Drawing the sample from one college of nursing was a limitation of this study, but Schriner used multiple methods of interview, document review, and observation. Schriner found that the values of the clinical practice role differed from values important for success in an academic faculty role. Often, the values and skills for which nurse faculty are hired, judged, and rewarded do not match those of the academy. Data from the Schriner study identified that faculty are often hired because they have a particular clinical expertise, with little regard for their competency as teachers. While clinical competency and expertise are required for clinical teaching, the hierarchy of real reward in some academic environments is dependent on the faculty's acquisition of research funding. While master's-prepared clinicians are seen as experts in the clinical environment, the culture of the academic environment can require a doctorate to be competitive. Schriner suggests that nursing education needs to change its reward structure to ensure that clinical expertise is clearly valued in the academic environment.

A grounded theory study conducted by Duffy (2013) investigated the academic role of nurse faculty and its influence on the formation of a personal academic identity. The sample consisted of 14 faculty in the United Kingdom who had a minimum of five years of teaching experience in higher education. Data were gathered using in-depth interviews. Findings from the study led to the identification of seven themes that formed the framework for a conceptual model of identity formation consisting of five stages: pre-entry, reaffirming, surmounting, stabilizing, and actualizing. Duffy noted that many of the concepts derived from the findings were dynamic in nature and evolved over time as participants responded to changes in institutional structure and social practices. As challenges emerged from an educational structure, participants re-engaged in the transformative phases of the model; thus, progression was both linear and cyclical. It was noted by some participants that an early emphasis on functional skills and competency within the traditional nursing education model inhibited their transition into and assimilation with the higher education model. This incongruence between the values of nursing and the expected behaviors in academia can have a significant impact on role development of nurse faculty. To make sense of the incongruence of the nursing values of nurturing and caring with those of academia, Duffy described three core identities: nursing, academic, and hybrid. Those who adopted a hybrid or academic identity reported greater assimilation with their role in the higher education environment. In addition, the study identified a need to balance academic and professional drivers, along with strategies such as experiential learning, seeking out role models, and informal support networks. Variation in self-confidence and engagement in the academic community signaled a need for ongoing support and professional development.

While little empirical evidence was found related to the integration of the mission of the institution in the work of nurse educators, both Schriner's (2007) and Duffy's (2013) findings illustrate the importance of the importance of "fit" with both the academic faculty role and the institution's mission. Alignment with the mission in the areas of faculty role, promotion and tenure, curriculum, and service is essential.

Strategically Responding to Trends in Higher Education

Higher education has faced many challenges over the past several years including greater economic pressures, evolving faculty roles and governance structures, and changing educational delivery systems. Most of these challenges are the result of externally driven pressures. "The conflict between the traditional autonomy of the scholar and demands for accountability to a variety of internal and external constituencies is one of the central issues of contemporary American higher education" (Bastedo, Altbach, & Gumport, 2016, p. 91). To successfully navigate today's increasingly complex educational environment and thrive in that environment, faculty need to be aware of social, economic, and political forces. Most of the literature in this area is not empirically based. Where gaps exist, nondatabased literature is presented to provide context and to identify research priorities for the future.

The landscape of the modern university continues to change with expanded access and increased diversity. In addition, universities face decreasing funding and greater oversight. These features have prompted changes in curricula and approaches to the delivery of knowledge, such as online learning and the use of information technologies in the classroom. There has also been a demand for greater transparency and accountability from consumers, as well as accrediting agencies. These trends have led to a focus on faculty roles, the intensity of academic work, and the impact on stress and work-life balance for faculty (Meyer, 2012).

Economic Pressures

Higher education has been economically affected by enrollment expansion, the Great Recession, changes in public spending priorities, and dwindling state support (Bastedo, Altbach, & Gumport, 2016). The cost of higher education and the resulting student indebtedness have been a stimulus for critical discourse in the United States. Students emerge from college with significant debt that affects their quality of life as they enter their new professional roles. The Center on Budget and Policy Priorities (2016) reported that the average state was spending 18 percent less per student on higher education than before the recession. The center also reported that public college tuition rates had risen by 33 percent since 2007, with one state reporting as high as a 90 percent increase. Despite tuition increases, the result has been faculty position cuts, eliminated course offerings, closed campuses, and reduced student services. At the same time, external pressures have resulted in a demand for greater accountability for student outcomes, transparency, and responsivity to meeting workforce needs.

In 2006, the Spellings report presented the findings and recommendations of the Commission on the Future of Higher Education (US Department of Education, 2006). To address the need for greater accountability and transparency, the commission recommended the development of a consumer-friendly database on higher education to enable stakeholders to compare institutions. In response to this recommendation, President Obama in 2013 announced a new college scorecard that provided data about tuition, graduation rates, and the average income of alumni (Neuman, 2017). In 2015, data on student debt and federal student loan repayment rates were added to that database (US Department of Education, 2016).

Nursing education has also felt the effects of external economic pressures. The financial effects of the Great Recession affected the ability of nursing schools to prepare enough nurses for workforce needs. Terry and Whitman (2011) conducted a study of 24 nursing deans or program directors from schools in the Southeast to examine the impact of the economic downturn on nursing schools in 2009–2010. Most respondents indicated that new-graduate employment recruitment had decreased (54.2 percent), undergraduate student applications increased (60.9 percent), graduate student applications increased (56.5 percent), and there was no change in faculty applicants (50 percent). Despite the increased number of student applications, the majority of deans or program directors (75 percent) said they were not going to accept more students. The major reason given for not accepting more applicants was the inability to place students for clinical education due to a lack of preceptors (25 percent) and inadequate clinical facilities (25 percent).

Nurse educators must consider the impact of curricular decisions and planning on students' financial outcomes. The Institute of Medicine (IOM, 2011) recommended the creation of seamless academic progression plans for nurses to achieve higher levels of academic progression. Curricula should be intentionally designed to facilitate this progression at both the undergraduate and graduate levels.

Evolving Faculty Roles and Governance

The expected role and function of the academic faculty member in higher education are often contextually dependent. These contexts are overlapping, including disciplinary, departmental, and institutional (Meyer, 2012). In addition, the academic faculty role in the environment of higher education can vary significantly by type of institution, location of the institution, program type, and department culture. The faculty role may consist of a combination of teaching and practical supervision, research and scholarship, and service to the university, the community, and the profession. An individual faculty role would typically be defined by the assigned percent of effort or time allocated to each of these areas.

To reduce costs and increase their financial flexibility, academic institutions have increasingly relied on contingent (adjunct) and non–tenure-track faculty to fill their teaching needs. Non–tenure-track faculty make up approximately 70 percent of all faculty nationally (Kezar & Maxey, 2013). They often lack the autonomy afforded to those on the tenure track and are given heavier teaching loads with less compensation. Contingent faculty lack employment protection, generally have low wages, and often do not participate in curricular planning. Most faculty face increased teaching workloads, either internally mandated or state mandated to control costs.

Many faculty are required to take on administrative functions in this new academic environment. "Academic planning, traditionally far removed from the individual professor and seldom impinging on academic careers, has become more of a reality as institutions seek to streamline their operations and worry more about external measures of productivity" (Bastedo et al., 2016, p. 100). The pressure for publication and research in some institutions has also intensified in the last two decades. With the decline in external funding sources for research, competition has increased (Bastedo et al., 2016).

Faculty Role Issues. Historically, the faculty role has included the tripartite of research, scholarship, and service within a tenure-earning model. However, the role of faculty today is much different with a fundamental shift of the academic workforce into mostly non–tenure-track positions that have been unbundled into teaching, research, or service-only roles. According to the Council for Higher Education Accreditation (CHEA, 2014), the nature of the academic workforce has fundamentally shifted over the last 40 years. Full-time tenured and tenure-track faculty were once the norm, whereas the professoriate of today consists mostly of non–tenure-track faculty. In 1969, tenured and tenure-track positions were 78.3 percent and nontenure positions were 21.7 percent of all positions. As of 2009, those figures had switched, with tenure and tenure-track positions decreasing to 33.5 percent and non–tenure-track positions increasing to 66.5 percent. The trend to shift to more full-time, non–tenure-track and part-time faculty is projected to continue (CHEA, 2014).

Evidence from the nursing literature suggests nurse faculty are experiencing workload strain related to increasing faculty role requirements. The nursing faculty shortage and role requirements (i.e., research/scholarship, teaching, service, practice, administration) have been demonstrated to contribute to faculty dissatisfaction. Smeltzer et al. (2016) examined the institutional features to maintain research productivity and analyzed predictors of productivity of 554 faculty teaching in nursing doctoral programs from 71 schools across the United States. They found that 60.6 percent of their respondents reported spending 16 or more hours a week in teaching classes. Clinical practice was also an element of workload for 34.5 percent; the majority of those engaged in clinical practice (54.3 percent) were teaching exclusively in DNP programs. The strongest predictor of research productivity was the average number of hours spent on research/scholarship-related activities ($\beta = .296$, $p < .001$) followed by time buy-out ($\beta = .270$, $p < .001$). In a subsequent publication, Smeltzer, Sharts-Hopko, Cantrell, Heverly, and Jenkinson (2017) did a content analysis of the qualitative data collected in the original study. Participants described workload concerns surrounding the impact of senior faculty retirements, a lack of workload credit for dissertation or capstone work, tenure-track requirements, work-life balance, time for scholarship, faculty shortages, and administrative responsibilities. Additionally, workload concerns of faculty teaching in all doctoral programs included multiple role responsibilities, too many students for faculty to manage, and the need to practice to maintain certification as an advanced practice nurse.

Faculty practice in nursing is an issue that has implications not only for overall workload consideration and balance but also for promotion and tenure. Becker et al. (2007) examined faculty practice using four focus groups composed of 46 full-time faculty from a single school in Maryland. They also completed individual interviews with the leaders from that school, as well as external interviews with leaders from nine additional schools of nursing across the United States. Their findings from the faculty focus groups revealed frustration with changing promotion and tenure criteria regarding the scholarship of practice and role strain and tension associated with the competing demands of practice, teaching, scholarship, and service. The researchers recommended that faculty carefully analyze their time spent in clinical practice and clinical teaching and ensure that these are reflected in their workloads. An additional recommendation was for promotion and tenure committees to "clearly define and differentiate the scholarship of practice" (Becker et al., 2007, p. 54).

In 2012, Pohl, Duderstadt, Tolve-Schoeneberger, Uphold, and Thorman Hartig reported on the findings of the National Organization of Nurse Practitioner Faculties (NONPF) Faculty Practice Survey regarding promotion and tenure. They found that more than half (51 percent) of those responding reported that practice was not a consideration in promotion and/or tenure decisions; similarly, 51 percent reported insufficient resources to support the mission of faculty practice. Significant predictors of successfully achieving promotion and tenure were the following: practice being considered in promotion and tenure ($p < .01$) and school level of support for practice ($p < .05$). Receiving school of nursing support increased the odds of being granted tenure by more than 1.5 times (odds ratio = 1.6). Nicholes and Dyer (2012) also examined perspectives and practices regarding tenure and DNP-prepared faculty in a sample of 65 faculty and administrators. The majority of the sample reported that DNP faculty were eligible for tenure in their institutions (61.3 percent, $n = 38$) and that practice was not considered for tenure (56.25 percent, $n = 36$).

Nurse educators must carefully consider the promotion and tenure policies and workload practices of potential places of employment. A mismatch in expectations could result in dissatisfaction with the faculty role and attrition. Clinical practice, which is essential for continued certification and competence, must be considered as part of the faculty role through supportive faculty practice plans. Faculty engagement in shared governance processes can ensure that they play an important role in helping to shape these practices and policies.

Faculty Governance Issues. Faculty governance, a long-standing structure of colleges and universities, has been faced with some new challenges. A survey by the Association of Governing Boards (AGB, 2016) of 300 college presidents and 2,250 governing board members found that over 50 percent of both groups said shared governance should function as a system of aligning priorities. However, only 33 percent of the governing board members and 25 percent of presidents said that their governance structures function in that way. The authors reported that there is often reduced capacity for faculty to serve in faculty governance roles because of the increasing numbers of non–tenure-track and contingent faculty.

There are multiple indicators that faculty in US colleges and universities have been losing their historic prerogatives, including the most defining characteristic of tenure. In an analysis of data from the 2007–2008 Changing Academic Profession (CAP) survey, Finkelstein and Cummings (2012) compared US faculty to faculty contemporaries in the 19 countries that participated in the study. For this analysis, the researchers examined the following aspects of institutional life: the faculty role in institutional governance, who evaluates the faculty's teaching and research, the placement of faculty loyalties between their academic departments and their institutions, and career and job satisfaction. Finkelstein and Cummings (2012) found that fewer than one tenth of US faculty reported a decisive role in selecting administrators and establishing budget priorities, and fewer than one third reported a decisive role in establishing new academic programs. On the other hand, more than half reported a decisive role in the appointment and promotion of academic staff. Findings related to the evaluation of teaching and research indicated that there is a powerful and pervasive role of students in the evaluation of teaching, both in the United States and other countries. Additionally, 50 percent of US faculty reported that other faculty were involved in evaluating their teaching, which was higher than in other English-speaking countries. Deans and directors were reported to have pervasive involvement in the evaluation of teaching by 80 percent of US faculty. Despite the trends of increased non-tenure-earning positions and the unbundling of the faculty role, the data revealed that US faculty perceived a relatively well-developed infrastructure for academia in the United States (Finkelstein & Cummings, 2012).

While faculty governance structures exist, faculty are often disengaged. Kater (2017) conducted a qualitative embedded multicase study of 27 faculty leaders in governance from nine community colleges to describe their perceptions of shared governance. Apathy and faculty disengagement in shared governance emerged as a theme from the data. Kater suggested that the corporatization of community colleges, heavy workloads, and a large percentage of adjunct faculty are factors that influence a lack of faculty participation and interest in shared governance.

Little was found in the empirical literature about nursing faculty governance. Boswell, Opton, and Owen (2016) published a literature review on shared governance in nursing using the key terms job satisfaction, empowerment, and work engagement in the academic setting. The researchers chose these search terms as they were found to be consistent with the existence of shared governance. They found that most of the nursing literature on shared governance was practice related and could not be applied to the academic setting. Job satisfaction was found to be an outcome of shared governance, and empowerment was a key factor in attaining job satisfaction. Transparency and ease of communication were found to be essential for the implementation of shared governance. Most significantly, Boswell et al. reported that empowerment was key to attaining organizational outcomes.

One case study was found that provides an illustration of the effects of the use of a governance process in a nursing program. Fontaine, Stotts, Saxe, and Scott (2008) published a case study on the use of a decision-making framework using shared faculty governance. The case involved faculty decision-making regarding possible implementation of a DNP program with data collection, analysis, and decision-making described within the context of shared governance. The authors stated that the participatory role of administration, rather than decision-making, critical analysis, and involvement by faculty, was a benefit of this model of decision-making. They also suggested that this model should be considered by other institutions, particularly when making high-stakes decisions.

Nurse educators need to be engaged in faculty governance both at the school/department level and at the overall university/college/school level. The level of engagement can vary, from awareness to leadership in faculty governance. Without engagement, a faculty member is surrendering the right to informed participative decision-making. As shared governance has been associated with empowerment and job satisfaction, nurse educators should carefully consider the extent to which shared governance plays a role in decision-making in potential places of employment.

Changing Educational Delivery Systems

As state budget appropriations and student grants have dwindled while costs have risen, higher education institutions have responded by making significant changes to their structures and processes, which has had a major impact on the work of faculty. Curricula are being examined and redesigned to maximize efficiency and minimize student credit hours. The value of a liberal education as an essential element of a college education has been challenged and minimized at some institutions. In other instances state legislatures have mandated that public institutions decrease the time to completion of a degree by reducing the number of credits required and minimizing the general education courses that all students must take. Competency-based education programs have emerged where students get credit for prior experience and move through their course of study at their own pace (Gravina, 2017).

One of the most significant strategies that higher education institutions have implemented is maximizing student enrollment by expanding the scope of educational offerings and targeting recruitment populations through distance education. In 2006, a rule that restricted federal financial aid for distance education was removed by Congress (US Department of Education, 2016). This opened the door for tremendous growth in this market. The most recent statistics from the National Center for Education Statistics (NCES) indicated that in 2011–2012, 36 percent of undergraduate and 36 percent of graduate students took distance education classes. Six percent of undergraduate and 18 percent of graduate students completed their entire degree program via distance education. These percentages have increased from previous years (NCES, 2015). Resulting from this expanded reach, institutional competition for students has become national or international, rather than the traditional regional competitive base. Students can now shop for programs that meet their individual needs from a much wider range of options.

Despite the rapid adoption of distance education programs, concerns still exist about student attrition, particularly in entirely online programs (Bawa, 2016). Essential to student retention and completion of a distance education program is student engagement. Faculty have had to become proficient in online teaching, which requires a different skill set than the traditional in-class teaching role. Successfully delivering distance education programs is resource intensive and requires faculty development and buy-in by faculty.

Distance education has taken on a significant role in nursing education nationally, in both undergraduate and graduate programs. Mancuso (2009) completed an integrative literature review of faculty perceptions of distance education in nursing. The studies reviewed reported increased faculty workload associated with distance education; difficulty transitioning to a different type of teaching role, from content delivery to facilitator; and the benefits of teaching online, which included flexibility and convenience. Faculty development, including instructional design, technology, and teaching strategies, as well as mentoring and ongoing support, was essential to student success and faculty satisfaction.

Consideration of the faculty role when teaching from a distance is of interest to nursing education. Goodfellow, Zungolow, Lockhart, Turk, and Dean (2014) published a case study of a distant faculty model. The purpose of the case study was to evaluate the impact of the model on the faculty member and the organization. The model included teaching, scholarship, and service within the context of presence. Goodfellow et al. found that the faculty member met and at times exceeded expectations in all areas. They concluded that given organizational structures and processes to support faculty engagement at a distance, this can be a viable model for future distant faculty appointments.

Engagement is a challenge in distance education environments. Smith and Crowe (2017) qualitatively examined nurse educators' perceptions of the importance of relationships in online teaching and learning. Ten nurse educators from across the United States were interviewed. Smith and Crowe found that "that there was an interconnected nature among (a) student engagement and learning, (b) 'knowing students,' and (c) supporting students in meeting their own needs" (Smith & Crowe, 2017, p. 13). The researchers described a connection between the relationship between the faculty and the student and engagement and cited this as a challenge for faculty at a distance.

Nurse educators face many challenges in transitioning to teaching in distance education environments. Gazza (2017) used a hermeneutic phenomenologic approach to understand the lived experience of teaching online in nursing education among 14 nurse faculty. Emerging from the data were four themes: "(a) Looking at a Lot of Moving Parts, (b) Always Learning New Things, (c) Going Back and Forth, and (d) Time Is a Blessing and a Curse" (p. 345). The findings described a learning environment that required a significant time and engagement commitment to be successful. Similar to previous studies, support was found to be essential for success.

Distance education is an educational trend that has grown over time, and nursing education has embraced this delivery method for all levels of nursing education. Nurse educators need to consider if the distance education environment is a fit for their teaching style and be prepared to design an engaging and effective educational experience for students in online learning environments. Faculty who teach online need to develop competencies in both the use of technology in the teaching/learning process and online student engagement skills to help students achieve their learning outcomes. Nurse educators should ensure that they have the support systems needed in their institutions to ensure their success.

Collaborating with Internal and External Constituents

Another theme related to functioning within the educational environment that was found in this literature review was the need for nurse faculty to collaborate with internal and external constituents. Little empirical literature was found regarding the nurse educator's role in collaboration; however, there has been a significant call for academic-practice partnerships that may provide direction for future research. To enhance nursing's influence within the academic community, faculty need to engage in strategic, multilevel partnerships with local, state, and national organizations and interdisciplinary networks. The goal is to develop innovative ways to communicate and work together on projects that address the needs of nursing and health care.

Nursing plays a critical role in the delivery of health care. The IOM (2011) *Future of Nursing* report recommended that nurses achieve higher levels of education and training through an improved education system that promotes seamless academic progression. To ensure a robust educational system that can meet this challenge, collaboration between nursing education and practice is essential.

To identify how to best position nursing schools for long-term success and sustainability, the American Association of Colleges of Nursing (AACN, 2016) commissioned a comprehensive study to identify strategies to support partnerships between academic nursing and academic health centers. Interviews were conducted with a variety of stakeholders affiliated with Academic Health Centers (AHCs) and non-AHC institutions. Findings from these interviews were discussion points for a national summit of AHC leaders. In addition, two surveys were issued to AHC leaders. The insights and understanding gained through these activities culminated in a report titled *Advancing Healthcare Transformation: A New Era for Academic Nursing* (the Manatt Report; AACN, 2016).

The AACN report (2016) addressed how baccalaureate and higher degree schools of nursing can strengthen their efforts to improve health care at the local, state, and national levels. It recommended six actions for institutional leaders: embrace a new vision for academic nursing; enhance the clinical practice of academic nursing; partner in preparing the nurses of the future; partner in the implementation of accountable care; invest in nursing research programs and better integrate research into clinical practice; and implement an advocacy agenda to support a new era for academic nursing. The findings were clear that an enhanced partnership with academic nursing is essential to an integrated transformation of health care. This transformation is dependent on academic faculty engagement at local, state, and national levels.

The interdependence of academic nursing and the service sector must be understood and appreciated by both. Each must steer away from a history of segregated resources and cooperatively embrace interrelated challenges with an appreciation for the policy and political implications of such academic-service partnerships.

While the AACN (2016) addressed baccalaureate and higher degree schools of nursing, community college and associate degree schools of nursing have also been engaged in strategic partnerships addressing the national priority of advancing the educational preparation of RNs to the baccalaureate level. Community colleges and collaborating universities have engaged in academic partnerships to develop and implement seamless, low-cost opportunities for RNs to achieve a BSN. Knowlton and Angel (2017) described one such partnership: the Regionally Increasing Baccalaureate Nurses (RIBN) Program. The authors described the experience of a collaboration that began as an academic partnership between one community college and one regional university that evolved to include 39 different academic institutions in partnerships across the state of North Carolina.

Warner and Burton (2009), in their report of a collaborative between the University of Portland (UP) and Providence Health and Services (PHS) resulting in the development of a dedicated education unit (DEU), contend that new thinking and changes are required for partnership models. The authors outlined the traditional approach of segregated and siloed allocation of resources, contrasted against a new model of academic-service partnerships. The DEU, presented as an exemplar of an academic-service partnership, is described as a client unit delivering quality patient care that serves as a "home-base," positive clinical learning environment where staff nurses, who serve as clinical instructors, receive support from an academic partner. Because in the UP-PHS model there was exclusive use of the DEU by one school, the staff nurses understood program outcomes, shared ownership in the curriculum, and had a deep investment in the formation of the nursing students.

According to Warner and Burton (2009), such partnerships signal a new way of thinking about the challenges that face nursing workforce development. The politics required for this new thinking involve letting go, accepting, and shifting to allow resources to be allocated creatively and with greater efficiency. The authors noted that this model has since been widely disseminated as a solution to "redistribute faculty workload, create a more intense and practice-grounded student experience, and enable schools to enroll more students" (Warner & Burton, 2009, p. 330).

As noted, collaborations evolve within variable economic and political contexts. Therefore, nurse educators in all educational settings must endeavor to remain current on public policy related to health care and higher education. Further, they must engage with the professional associations leading efforts in this regard. Such organizations as the NLN, the AACN, and the National Organization of Nurse Practitioner Faculty (NONPF) work with legislators and regulators on behalf of nursing and nursing faculty.

Creating a Collegial Environment

A sense of collegiality has been identified by numerous sources as a significant factor for ensuring a healthy work environment in the academic setting (Clark, 2013; McDonald, 2010; NLN, 2006; Peters, 2014; Tourangeau et al., 2013). Connecting to academia with a sense of belonging is vital for developing competence in the nurse faculty role. McDonald (2010) performed a review of the literature regarding new-nurse faculty transition and identified three themes: knowledge deficit, salary and workload, and culture and support. The theme of culture and support identified the importance of faculty fitting into a new culture. Along with mentoring, McDonald found that camaraderie among new faculty helped create a good support system.

Tourangeau et al. (2013) employed a cross-sectional survey designed to identify the variables that influence nurse faculty's intention to remain (ITR) employed in an academic setting. The sample included 650 Ontario (Canada) nurse faculty. Ten of 26 independent variables explained 25.4 percent of the variance in nurse faculty ITR for five years. The "quality of relationships with colleagues" was one of the influencing factors. Findings from this study highlighted the importance of implementing strategies that support collegial relationships among faculty.

Although collegiality has been identified as the goal, faculty may experience negative or confrontational interactions with other faculty. Incivility can create significant challenges to achieving a collegial academic environment. It is important for faculty to prepare themselves to cope with or learn strategies to defend against situations of faculty-to-faculty incivility. Peters (2014) studied novice nurse faculty members' lived experience of faculty-to-faculty incivility. The purposive sample consisted of eight faculty with less than five years of experience. Five themes emerged: sensing rejection, employing behaviors to cope with uncivil colleagues, sensing others wanted novice faculty to fail, sensing a possessiveness of territory from senior faculty, and struggling with the decision to remain in the faculty position. Peters warned that allowing uncivil behaviors to go unaddressed may negatively impact nursing education. This study highlighted the importance of mentoring and supporting collegiality as a means to achieve a healthy academic work environment.

Clark (2013) conducted a mixed-methods study to describe faculty-to-faculty incivility. The sample consisted of 588 nurse faculty from 40 US states and was not confined to novice faculty. The median number of years in teaching was 10 years (range from less than 1 year to 40 years). The qualitative portion of the study sought to identify how faculty described uncivil faculty-to-faculty encounters, as well as effective ways to address incivility. Eight themes emerged to describe uncivil encounters: "berating, insulting, and allowing; setting up, undermining and sabotaging; power playing, derailing, and disgracing; excluding, gossiping, and degrading; refusing, not doing, and justifying; blaming and accusing; taking credit (ripping off) the work of others; distracting and disrupting during meetings" (p. 99). Six themes emerged to describe strategies to foster civility and collegiality: "direct communication between and among faculty; installing and sustaining effective, competent leadership; measuring incivility and implementing policies and protocols; education faculty, and raising awareness; transforming the organizational culture; and building and fostering faculty relationships and collaborations" (p. 101).

Clark (2013) pointed out that dealing with incivility takes personal courage. While respondents expressed anger and frustration that incivility was tolerated and often ignored, many expressed reluctance to address it themselves. Many respondents in the Clark study expressed fear of retaliation or lack of confidence in their skills of confrontation. Clark advised that critical conversations need to be approached purposefully and thoughtfully, noting that the ultimate goal is to develop personal relationships and build professional collaborations to foster a culture of collegiality.

Incivility presents a significant challenge to the maintenance of a healthy work environment in academia. Schools of nursing have an obligation to support healthy work environments. The NLN (2006) examined work environments in academia and published the Healthful Work Environment Tool Kit (http://nln.org/professional-development-programs/teaching-resources/toolkits/healthful-work-environment), designed as a tool for nurse faculty to strategically examine their work environment, engage stakeholders, and develop an action plan to support a healthful work environment. Belonging to such a community of practice with a healthy work environment has a significant influence on the faculty experience.

Leading the Way

The final theme that emerged from the literature review was the faculty role as leader. Leadership is broadly defined as both informal and formal leadership within an institution, as well as within the profession. The empirical evidence regarding nurse faculty leadership has been primarily qualitative and reflects experiences, perspectives, competencies, and desired qualities. What is not evident in the literature is the connection between leadership and academic outcomes, such as faculty satisfaction and the work environment.

In a series of reports emerging from data collected from 21 faculty leaders in nursing education using interpretive phenomenology (Young, Pearsall, Stiles, Nelson, & Horton-Deutsch, 2011), several themes emerged in relation to their leadership experience. Young et al. reported that faculty leaders were thrust into leadership, neither seeking nor being prepared for early leadership roles. The researchers found that leaders took risks in their teaching and in their faculty role. All shared the challenge of building consensus among other faculty. Stiles, Pardue, Young, and Morales (2011) reported on the theme of advancing educational reform, with faculty being involved with others, struggling to serve as symbols and preserve authenticity, and creating an environment for change. In the most recent report, Pearsall et al. (2014) reported on the hermeneutic analysis of data from 14 of the same nurse faculty participants, including two focus group narratives on the meaning of taking a risk for leadership development. Emerging from the data were four themes: "doing their homework to minimize risk-taking, weighing the costs and benefits, learning the context, and cultivating relationships" (Pearsall et al., 2014, p. 27). Risk-taking both within and outside the organization was found to be an essential element of faculty leadership.

Kalb, O'Conner-Von, Schipper, Watkins, and Yetter (2012) explored faculty perspectives in educating leaders in nursing among 76 faculty teaching in associate, bachelor's, master's, and practice doctorate programs in a single academic institution using qualitative analysis obtained from a researcher-designed survey. The first theme that emerged from their analysis was the commitment of faculty to engage in self-development as leaders in nursing. Important to that development was being passionate about nursing, engaging in self-reflection and knowing self, and serving others, including participation in professional nursing organizations.

In 2015, Patterson and Krouse identified competencies of leaders in nursing education from a descriptive analysis of interview data from 15 nursing education leaders in all parts of the United States. The competencies that were identified included articulate and promote a vision for nursing education; function as a steward for the organization and nursing education; embrace, articulate, and promote a vision for nursing education; embrace professional values in the context of higher education; and develop and nurture relationships.

Delgado and Mitchell (2017) reported on findings from 52 nurse educators from 12 different US schools on the most valued qualities of academic leadership in nursing. The survey, developed by the researchers, asked participants to rank items from most to least important. The most important characteristics, in rank order, were integrity, clarity in communication, and problem-solving ability.

Nurse educators need to be prepared to become leaders as faculty members, to assume both formal and informal leadership roles in academia. Formal leadership development programs should focus on the development of the competencies for leaders in nursing education identified in the literature. Additionally, faculty should be prepared to successfully overcome the challenges reflected in these studies. Leaders in nursing education have the responsibility of advancing the nursing profession through their influence on national and international nursing and health care issues.

Political Advocacy

Little evidence was found in the literature regarding faculty engagement in external advocacy activities, including policy and politics. A literature search revealed calls to action, particularly regarding health care reform and professional licensing issues. Hewlett, Bleich, Cox, and Hoover (2009), in their call to action, also found a gap in the literature in this area. They stated this is of significant concern because "nurses are not often noted as a powerful, knowledgeable, or entrepreneurial entity in the world of educational system policy and politics" (p. 324).

The limited empirical evidence that was found regarding the faculty role in political advocacy was embedded in a study of practices, perceptions, and barriers to teaching health policy by Staebler et al. (2017). The researchers sent an online invitation to all AACN nurse faculty members across the United States and received 514 completed surveys. They reported that 70.5 percent of respondents who taught health policy reported experiences advocating for nursing within health care and policy communities. Only 44.3 percent were active in legislative advocacy. One third of the respondents reported that in their schools, policy content in the curriculum was not an important priority. More than 50 percent of the faculty cited a lack of desire, and 49.1 percent reported a lack of opportunity as barriers to faculty development in advocacy and policy expertise.

IDENTIFIED GAPS IN THE LITERATURE

Empirical evidence in the nursing education literature for many of the elements of this nurse educator competency is minimal. Quantitative studies reported in the literature have focused on the changing role and function of nurse educators and the impact on job satisfaction and retention. Qualitative inquiry has focused on the experiences of nurse educators, particularly novice faculty, regarding socialization and acculturation during initial transition to the faculty role.

Collegiality is known to foster a healthy work environment conducive to the academic enterprise making it possible to achieve the dual mission of creating new knowledge through research and disseminating knowledge through teaching. Although much attention has been spent on the issues of incivility and healthful work environments, there has been little empirical study to develop evidence-based strategies to combat incivility or evidence-based interventions to support increased collegiality.

This nurse educator competency also calls for nurse educators to be engaged in shared governance within the institution and become voices for nursing education in engagement with external constituencies. While some empirical evidence exists in higher education literature regarding faculty engagement and the impact of shared governance in higher education, there is very little about faculty engagement and its impact on shared governance. This is of increasing concern because of the proliferation of distance education. Nurse educators may not have a physical presence on campus, and current nursing practice requirements may not fit well with the traditional faculty model. A disrupter in nursing education has been the DNP degree. While there exists some evidence as to how nurse educators with this degree are currently being integrated into academia, there is no evidence regarding role satisfaction, attrition, and outcomes.

There is concern regarding the growing workload of nurse educators in academia and the impact of practice requirements on both workload and promotion and tenure. While some evidence exists regarding the impact of practice requirements on nurse educators and the integration of practice into the faculty role, there is no evidence that has examined the impact of practice requirements on faculty attrition and role satisfaction. No literature was found regarding faculty engagement in political discourse in the areas of health policy and nursing education or strategies to engage faculty. While evidence of structured opportunities for faculty engagement in advocacy for policy issues was found among the professional nursing education organizations (AACN, NLN), there was no evidence that described the level of engagement in those activities.

PRIORITIES FOR FUTURE RESEARCH

Research is needed to further understand and articulate the expectations for the role of the nurse educator in academia, examine how the context of the higher education environment specifically influences the nurse educator, and determine how to create the most favorable work environment for nurse educators. The concept of incivility needs to be more comprehensively investigated at all levels where these interactions occur and have the potential to disrupt faculty relationships and the learning environment.

Investigation is needed to develop an understanding of what factors attract and support retention of nurse educators, including how to support the connection between faculty strengths and the program mission. Research is also needed to understand the effects of changing economic, legislative, and political influences on the nurse educator as they relate to fulfilling the educator's role and function. Further, the nurse educator's role with regard to engagement in collaborations, partnerships, legislative policy, and politics needs to be more empirically studied. These areas of research are essential to more fully understand and expand faculty capacity for the following competencies where little empirical evidence currently exists: incorporates the goals of the nursing program and the mission of the parent institution when proposing change or managing issues, assumes a leadership role in various levels of institutional governance, and advocates for nursing and nursing education in the political arena (NLN, 2012).

Areas for future research include, but are not limited to, the following:

▸ What faculty workload and practice models are most effective based on institutional mission?

▸ What is the impact of faculty workload and practice requirements on promotion and tenure and intent to stay in the academic environment?

▸ What are the most effective strategies by which to overcome faculty-to-faculty incivility and support collegiality?

▸ How can nurse educators be engaged in political action and policy development, and what is the impact on student policy engagement?

▸ What is the relationship between academic leadership and faculty recruitment/competence/satisfaction/retention?

▸ What models or measures are useful in assessing the impact of academic-practice and academic-service partnerships?

References

American Association of Colleges of Nursing. (2016). *Advancing healthcare transformation: A new era for academic nursing.* Retrieved from http://www.aacnnursing.org/Portals/42/News/AACN-Manatt-Report.pdf?ver = 2017-04-27-093429-050

Association of Governing Boards. (2016). *Shared governance: Is OK good enough?* Retrieved from https://www.agb.org/reports/2016/shared-governance-is-ok-good-enough

Bastedo, M. N., Altbach, P. G., & Gumport, P. J. (Eds.). (2016). *American higher education in the 21st century: Social, political, and economic challenges* (4th ed.). Baltimore, MD: Johns Hopkins University Press.

Bawa, P. (2016, January-March). Retention in online courses: Exploring issues and solutions – A literature review. *Sage Open*, 1–11. doi:10.1177/2158244015621777

Becker, K. L., Dang, D., Jordan, E., Kub, J., Welch, A., Smith, C. A., & White, K. M. (2007). An evaluation framework for faculty practice. *Nursing Outlook*, 55, 44–54. doi:10.1016/j.outlook.2006.10.001

Boswell, C., Opton, L., & Owen, D. (2016). Exploring shared governance for an academic nursing setting. *Journal of Nursing Education, 56,* 197–203. doi:10.3928/01484834-20170323-02

Center on Budget and Policy Priorities. (2016). *Education department proposes rule on state authorization of post-secondary distance education, foreign locations.* Retrieved from http://www.ed.gov/news/press-releases/education-department-proposes-rule-state-authorization-postsecondary-distance-education-foreign-locations

Council for Higher Education Accreditation. (2014). *An examination of the changing faculty: Ensuring institutional quality and achieving desired student learning outcomes.* Retrieved from https://www.chea.org/userfiles/Occasional%20Papers/Examination_Changing_Faculty_2013.pdf

Clark, C. (2013). National study on faculty-to-faculty incivility: Strategies to foster collegiality and civility. *Nurse Educator, 38,* 98–102.

Delgado, C., & Mitchell, M. M. (2017). A survey of current valued academic leadership qualities in nursing. *Nursing Education Perspectives, 37,* 10–15. doi:10.5480/14-1496

Duffy, R. (2013). Nurse to faculty? Academic roles and the formation of personal academic identities. *Nurse Education Today, 33,* 620–624. doi:10.1016/j.nedt.2012.07.020

Finkelstein, M., & Cummings, W. (2012). American faculty and their institutions: The global view. *Change Magazine,* 48–59. doi:10.1080/00091383.2012.672882

Fontaine, D., Stotts, N., Saxe, J., & Scott, M. (2008). Shared faculty governance: A decision-making framework for evaluating the DNP. *Nursing Outlook, 56,* 167–173. doi:10.1016/j.outlook.2008.02.008

Gazza, E. (2017). The experience of teaching online in nursing education. *Journal of Nursing Education, 56,* 343–349. doi:10.3928/01484834-20170518-05

Goodfellow, L., Zungolow, E., Lockhart, J. S., Turk, M., & Dean, B. (2014). Successes and challenges of a distant faculty model. *Nursing Forum, 49,* 288-29. doi:10.1111/nuf.12060

Gravina, E. W. (2017). Competency-based education and its effect on nursing education: A literature review. *Teaching and Learning in Nursing, 12,* 117–121. doi:10.1016/j.teln.2016.11.004

Hewlett, P. O., Bleich, M., Cox, M. F., & Hoover, K. W. (2009). Changing times: The role of academe in health reform. *Journal of Professional Nursing, 25,* 322–328. doi:10.1016/j.profnurs.2009.10.008

Institute of Medicine. (2011). *The future of nursing: Leading change, advancing health.* Washington, DC: National Academies Press.

Kalb, K. A., O'Conner-Von, S. K., Schipper, L. M., Watkins, A. K., & Yetter, D. M. (2012). Educating leaders in nursing: Faculty perspectives. *International Journal of Nursing Education Scholarship, 9,* 1–13. doi:10.1515/15 48–923X.2215

Kater, S. (2017). Community college faculty conceptualizations of shared governance: Shared understandings of a sociopolitical reality. *Community College Review, 45,* 234–257. doi:10.1177/0091552117700490

Kezar, A., & Maxey, D. (2013). The changing academic workforce. *Trusteeship, 21.* Retrieved from https://www.agb.org/trusteeship/2013/5/changing-academic-workforce

Knowlton, M. C., & Angel, L. (2017). Lessons learned: Answering the call to increase the BSN workforce. *Journal of Professional Nursing, 33*(3), 184–193. doi:10.1016/j.profnurs.2016.08.015

Mancuso, J. (2009). Perceptions of distance education among nursing faculty members in North America. *Nursing and Health Sciences, 11,* 194–205. doi:10.1111/j.1442-2018.2009.00456.x

McDonald, P. (2010). Transitioning from clinical practice to nursing faculty: Lessons learned. *Journal of Nursing Education, 49,* 126–131. doi:10.3928/01484834-20091022-02

Meyer, L. (2012). Negotiating academic values, professorial responsibilities and expectations for accountability in today's university. *Higher Education Quarterly, 66,* 207–217. doi:10.1111/j.1468-2273.2012.00516.x

National Center for Education Statistics (NCES). (2015). *Distance education in postsecondary institutions.* Retrieved from https://nces.ed.gov/programs/coe/indicator_sta.asp

National League for Nursing (NLN). (2006). *Healthful work environment tool kit.* Retrieved from http://www.nln.org/ professional-development-programs/ teaching-resources/toolkits/healthful- work-environment

National League for Nursing (NLN). (2012). *The scope of practice for academic nurse educators.* New York, NY: Author.

Neuman, W. R. (2017). Charting the future of US higher education: A look at the Spellings report ten years later. *Liberal Education, 103.* Retrieved from https://www.aacu.org/ liberaleducation/2017/winter/neuman

Nicholes, R. H., & Dyer, J. (2012). Is eligibility for tenure possible for the Doctor of Nursing Practice-prepared faculty? *Journal of Professional Nursing, 28,* 13–17. doi:10.1016/ j.profnurs.2011.10.001

Patterson, B. J., & Krouse, A. M. (2015). Competencies for leaders in nursing education. *Nursing Education Perspectives, 36,* 76–82. doi:10.5480/13-1300

Pearsall, C., Pardue, K. T., Horton-Deutsch, S., Young, P. K., Halstead, J., Nelson, K. A., … Zungolo, E. (2014). Becoming a nurse faculty leader: Doing your homework to minimize risk taking. *Journal of Professional Nursing, 30,* 26–33. doi:10.1016/j. profnurs.2012.10.010

Peters, A. (2014). Faculty to faculty incivility: Experiences of novice nurse faculty in academia. *Journal of Nursing, 30,* 213–227. doi:10.1016/jprofnurs.2013.09.007

Pohl, J. M., Duderstadt, K., Tolve- Schoeneberger, C., Uphold, C. R., & Thorman Hartig, M. (2012). Faculty practice: What do the data show? Findings from the NONPF faculty practice survey. *Nursing Outlook, 60*(5), 250–258. doi:10.1016/ j.outlook.2012.06.008

Schriner, C. (2007). The influence of culture on clinical nurses transitioning into the faculty role. *Nursing Education Perspectives, 28,* 145–149.

Smeltzer, S. C., Cantrell, M. A., Sharts-Hopko, N. C., Heverly, M. A., Jenkinson, A., & Nthenge, S. (2016). Assessment of the impact of teaching demands on research productivity among doctoral nursing program faculty. *Journal of Professional Nursing, 32,* 180–192. doi:10.1016/j. profnurs.2015.06.011

Smeltzer, S. C., Sharts-Hopko, N. C., Cantrell, M. A., Heverly, M. A., & Jenkinson, A. (2017). Nursing doctoral faculty perceptions related to the effect of increasing enrollments on productivity. *Nursing Education Perspectives, 38,* 201–202. doi:10.1097/01. NEP.0000000000000145

Smith, Y. M., & Crowe, A. R. (2017). Nurse educator perceptions of the importance of relationship in online teaching and learning. *Journal of Professional Nursing, 33,* 11–19. doi:10.1016/j.profnurs.2016.06.004

Staebler, S., Campbell, J., Cornelius, P., Fallin-Bennett, A., Fry-Bowers, E., Kung, Y. M., LaFevers, D.… (2017). Policy and political advocacy: Comparison study of nursing faculty to determine current practices, perceptions, and barriers to teaching health policy. *Journal of Professional Nursing, 33,* 350–355. doi:10.1016/j.profnurs.2017.04.001

Stiles, K., Pardue, K. T., Young, P., & Morales, M. L. (2011). Becoming a nurse faculty leader: Practices of leading illuminated through advancing reform in nursing education. *Nursing Forum, 46,* 94–101. doi:10.1111/j.1744-6198.2011.00214.x

Terry, A., & Whitman, M. V. (2011). Impact of the economic downturn on nursing schools. *Nursing Economic, 29,* 252–264.

Tourangeau, A., Saari, M., Patterson, E., Ferron, E., Thomson, H., Widger, K., & MacMillan, K. (2013). Work, work environments and other factors influencing nurse faculty intention to remain employed: A cross-sectional study. *Nurse Education Today, 34,* 940–947. doi:10.1016/j.nedt.2013.10.010.

US Department of Education. (2006). *A test of leadership: Charting the future of U.S. higher education.* Retrieved from https:// www2.ed.gov/about/bdscomm/list/ hiedfuture/reports/pre-pub-report.pdf

US Department of Education. (2016). *Fact sheet: Obama administration announces release of new scorecard data.* Retrieved from https://www.ed.gov/news/press-releases/ fact-sheet-obama-administration- announces-release-new-scorecard-data

Warner, J., & Burton, D. (2009). The policy and politics of emerging academic-service partnerships. *Journal of Professional Nursing, 6*, 329–334. doi:10.1016/j.profnurs.2009.10.00

Young, P. K., Pearsall, C., Stiles, K. A., Nelson, K. A., & Horton-Deutsch, S. (2011). Becoming a nurse faculty leader. *Nursing Education Perspectives, 32*, 222–228. doi:10.5480/1536-5026-32.4.222

11

The Future Role of the Nurse Educator

Judith A. Halstead, PhD, RN, ANEF, FAAN

Publication of the NLN Core Competencies of Nurse Educators© in 2005 was a seminal event in nursing education. The publication defines the complexity of the nurse educator role and tangibly identifies the evidence-based competencies and associated task statements that embody the role. Valiga (2007) found the NLN competencies for nurse educators to be "key to our continued success in preparing graduates who provide exquisite care, who make significant contributions to interdisciplinary collaborations, and who influence the future of the profession" (p. 173). She emphasized that the competencies provided "a foundational step in achieving excellence in nursing education" (p. 173).

Since publication, the core competencies have emerged as a framework to guide the preparation of a well-qualified nurse educator workforce, based on the premise that faculty who demonstrate the competencies in their educator role will facilitate achievement of student learning outcomes and ultimately influence the quality of care delivered to patients. More than a decade later, what evidence do we have that the core competencies influence and shape the role of the nurse educator and the quality of nursing education being delivered in our programs?

The systematic review of literature described in this book demonstrates that there is a growing body of research related to the NLN Core Competencies of Nurse Educators in academic settings. However, there also exists much opportunity to continue to design and implement a research agenda to further develop the core competency framework and validate the premise that nurse educators who demonstrate the core competencies in their practice positively influence student learning outcomes. As noted throughout the chapters in this book, many of the research questions that were identified in the first core competency publication (Halstead, 2007) remain relevant. New research questions have also been identified, reflecting evolving trends in nursing education. While research related to the nurse educator core competencies has increased, this updated literature review reveals some oversights in areas related to the nurse educator role that cut across multiple competencies. These are missed opportunities to enhance and strengthen the educator role and the quality of nursing education offered in our nursing programs.

The purpose of this chapter is to highlight these identified research gaps, propose a future research agenda designed to address the nurse educator role, and propose future directions for the nurse educator role that are needed to shape a relevant, contemporary nurse educator workforce. The reader is referred to the specific competency chapters in this book for a complete discussion of the research that was reported for each core competency.

CROSS-COMPETENCY RESEARCH GAPS

The chapters in this book continue the literature review on the nurse educator core competencies from where the first review (covering the years 1992–2004) ended, providing a focused, evidence-based review of literature for the period 2005 to 2017 for each individual core competency. The authors of this updated review also identify some thematic gaps in the research that are common across multiple competencies. For example, in their review of literature related to the competency *Facilitate Learning*, Caputi and Frank note that much of the research continues to be focused on self-reported *perceptions* of student or faculty satisfaction and *perceptions* of effectiveness of various teaching strategies, with a lack of attention to the impact on student learning outcomes. To facilitate future development of the nurse educator role in facilitating learning, the focus needs to shift away from perceptions of satisfaction or the effectiveness of various teaching strategies to the identification and development of measurable student learning outcomes that will prepare graduates to provide the exquisite patient care that Valiga (2007) referenced. In addition, Caputi and Frank stress that the research related to the educator's role in designing effective clinical learning environments remains almost exclusively focused on undergraduate education.

Luparell has similar findings in her literature review for the competency *Facilitate Learner Development and Socialization,* noting that the published research for this competency remains primarily focused on students and faculty in undergraduate programs. She also addresses the importance of student learning outcomes in the observation that the literature is lacking studies on how best to achieve learner socialization and develop professional identity comportment. Luparell raises the question of what student learning outcomes related to learner professional socialization and identity are most important and how to measure them effectively. Similar to Caputi and Frank, Luparell makes the point that nurse educators need to develop further competence in strategies that facilitate the achievement of identified student learner outcomes.

Similar observations are made by Spurlock and Mariani in their review of the literature related to the core competency *Use Assessment and Evaluation Strategies*. While some research areas focused on nursing student assessment and evaluation have started to emerge (e.g., high-stakes testing and simulation), overall, research related to assessment and evaluation remains quite limited and lacking in depth. This was also the case in the first review of literature covering the years 1992 to 2004. They further note that graduate education is woefully underrepresented in the research literature related to the nurse educator's use of assessment and evaluation strategies. Consistent with other chapter authors and based on their literature review, Spurlock and Mariani conclude with the observation that nurse educators know little about the competencies needed to effectively promote, measure, and evaluate the optimal achievement of student learning outcomes.

Scheckel and Hedrick-Erickson, in their chapter on the competency *Participate in Curriculum Design and Evaluation of Program Outcomes,* point out that evidence-based approaches to curriculum design and program outcome evaluation remain sparse, with the exception of the emergence of an increased number of systematic reviews within the years covered by this review (2005–2017). They also note once again that there is a lack of research on graduate curricula and program outcomes, with most research focused on undergraduate curricula.

In addition to the repeated observations that the majority of the research literature reviewed for this book was focused on undergraduate education and that there is a lack of attention to the impact of nurse educators on the achievement of student learning outcomes, there was one other commonly observed finding. The majority of the research reviewed lacks a system perspective in design. In their chapter, Spurlock and Mariani address the quality of research in nursing education. They recommend that nursing education move beyond underpowered, single-site research designs that rely on such subjective measures as self-reporting and the use of measures that lack sufficient validity and reliability, and work to strengthen the quality of statistical reporting.

SETTING A RESEARCH AGENDA FOR THE ROLE OF THE NURSE EDUCATOR

The thematic research gaps that emerged from this updated review of the literature can provide some direction for a future research agenda related to the nurse educator role. For those who are seeking an area of research in nursing education within which to build a body of work, this provides many possible opportunities within which to do so. The reader will find specific research questions related to each competency and its task statements in the respective chapters. In addition, many of the research questions identified in the first core competency review of literature (1992–2004) remain relevant over a decade later and should not be ignored. While some areas of research emerged in the updated review that were not evident in the previous literature review (e.g., faculty role in the use of simulation technology), it is striking how much of the core competency research literature continues to focus on attempts to answer the same research questions repeatedly through the use of single-site, descriptive studies.

The need to address nursing education, including the nurse educator role, from an educational systems perspective and across the academic continuum from undergraduate to graduate education is becoming increasingly critical. As noted previously, there is a consistent lack of attention to graduate education and the faculty and students who teach and learn in these programs in our research. What leads to this lack of attention to the nurse educator role and how it plays out in graduate nursing education? Does the emphasis on the preparation of clinical researchers in graduate nursing programs lead to an inadvertent oversight of research about the educator role in teaching effectively in these programs?

Regardless of the cause, the role of the nurse educator in graduate nursing education deserves closer attention. The profession is grappling with identifying the best means by which to prepare graduates of relatively new graduate degree programs (i.e., CNL, DNP) while also engaging in the development of a variety of academic progression models that rapidly move the learner from undergraduate learning experiences to graduate learning. Interdisciplinary curriculum models that require collaboration in integrating core curricular learning concepts and outcomes into curricula for multiple professions are continuing to emerge as well. The complexity of these various educational models and learning environments demands that nurse educators be expert in their role at the systems level and design programs with that perspective in mind. Our programs of research in nursing education need to reflect these growing realities and address the systems questions that are generated by these new models of learning.

Given the lack of emphasis in the research literature on the role of the educator in identifying and promoting student learning outcomes, it is important for future research agendas to include studies designed to investigate how nurse educators can influence the achievement of student learning outcomes. Nurse educators have an important responsibility to design curricula and learning experiences in environments that facilitate students' successful achievement of desired learning outcomes. Furthermore, the focus needs to go beyond how best to facilitate outcome achievement to increasing nurse educator competence in assessing and evaluating student achievement of the learning outcomes. Programs of research related to this topic are particularly needed.

In addition, the core competency *Participate in Curriculum Design and Evaluation of Program Outcomes* could be greatly enhanced by research efforts that are fueled through partnerships with interdisciplinary partners and clinical practice partners with the goal of linking outcomes achieved through interdisciplinary learning outcomes to patient outcomes. For example, the use of an interdisciplinary research design model that links desired student learning outcomes to desired patient outcomes, and the development of educational strategies by which to consistently measure the achievement of such outcomes, has the potential to improve the relevance of our educational programs by impacting patient care. The design of relevant curricula for today's health care environment demands interdisciplinary efforts in partnership with our clinical partners, and the nurse educator role in leading and advocating for these curricular efforts is a crucial one.

The development of nurse educators as leaders and advocates would benefit from further study and strengthen the influence of the nurse educator role in nursing and health care. Nurse educators are not just responsible for their own leadership development; they must also help develop the leadership competencies of the future leaders of our profession—our students—and must work to effectively build the pipeline for leadership succession in nursing education and the profession. In their chapter on the core competency *Function as a Change Agent and Leader*, Specht and Gordon indicate that while some progress has been made over the past decade in defining the importance of the role of the nurse educator as a change agent and leader, research remains limited about how to most effectively develop these competencies in the nurse educator role. As a future area of research, they specifically identify the need to attend to "nurse leader fatigue" and how it impacts nurse educators as a special concern.

The core competency of *Function Within the Educational Environment* yielded little research in this most recent review of literature conducted by Krouse and Fox. The changing economic, political, and legislative influences on the educational environment impact the nurse educator's role. What does the confluence of emerging issues mean for future nurse educators? How will the role change, and what will emerge as significant satisfiers for those individuals who choose to pursue careers as academic nurse educators? What models of academic-practice partnerships will prove most effective in producing quality graduates from our nursing programs, and how will these partnerships influence the role of the nurse educator? These are all areas deserving of future study.

The NLN Core Competencies for Nurse Educators can be used as a framework to develop programs of research related to the nurse educator role. This review of literature demonstrates that there is opportunity for further research on the use of the core competency model. The core competencies have been used to design faculty development programs, job descriptions, and graduate program curricula to prepare nurse educators and serve as the framework for the NLN Certified Nurse Educator examination. Are there variations in the applicability of the model across different academic environments? Does the acquisition of the core competencies vary with the educators' educational background, experience as educators, the institutional environment, or the program type within which they teach? Are select core competencies more relevant to novice educators in their initial years of teaching, leading to a gradual broadening of their attainment of the core competencies as their experience as educators grows? Do educators who are proficient in the core competencies provide better student learning environments that lead to greater achievement of student learning outcomes?

In their review of the research literature related to the core competency *Engage in Scholarship,* Patterson and McLaughlin raise the question: what does being a scholar of nursing education mean to an academic nurse educator? Patterson and McLaughlin note that since the 2007 published review of literature, there has been an increased focus on research outputs, such as publications, and strategies to positively impact the productivity of scholars. However, they note that the development of a science of nursing education, with an understanding of the role of the nurse educator in engaging in scholarship and research, remains limited and somewhat elusive. They therefore issue a call for the application of scholarship to teaching strategies and student learning outcomes.

A national agenda for research in nursing education, published by the NLN, has existed for a number of years. The American Association of Colleges of Nursing (AACN, 2018) recently published a task force consensus statement *Defining Scholarship for Academic Nursing*, which includes references to the scholarship of teaching. The consensus statement highlights examples of scholarship of teaching that emphasize systems design, outcome evaluation, and interprofessional education efforts designed to affect patient outcomes. These examples represent a radical departure from previous teaching scholarship efforts and have the potential to greatly impact the nurse educator role and how it is implemented.

One might raise the question of what impact the existence of a national research agenda on nursing education and other professional statements can have on developing the science of nursing education. Are there ways by which to measure the impact or to further leverage the existence of a national research agenda in developing the science of nursing education? What does it actually mean to develop the science of nursing education, especially as it relates to the role of the nurse educator? Determining specific goals and outcomes of research related to the educator role may be useful in further defining the nurse educator core competency model. With a targeted research agenda, mentoring, and focused calls for research proposals that only fund research with appropriate rigor in the research design, future directions for the nurse educator role can be developed that will benefit the quality of nursing education.

FUTURE DIRECTIONS FOR THE NURSE EDUCATOR ROLE

In Valiga's review of the literature relevant to the core competency of *Pursue Continuous Quality Improvement in the Nurse Educator Role,* she notes that a lack of preparation for the educator role continues to persist within the profession. With the nurse faculty shortage that the profession is experiencing and the lack of qualified individuals prepared to meet the demands of the role, one can assume that this situation will be ongoing for the foreseeable future. But can the profession afford to continue to neglect the preparation of nurse educators equipped with the requisite competencies needed to prepare nurses who can function effectively in changing environments?

The system complexities inherent in both health care and higher education, and the increasingly complex educational models that are being designed in our nursing schools, demand that the profession seriously consider how best to nurture a workforce of qualified nurse educators well versed and up-to-date in issues facing nursing, health care, and education. To achieve this, the nursing profession will need to acknowledge the value of preparing nurses who desire an academic career with expertise in nursing education. Continuing to deny this as a relevant need is detrimental to the quality of nursing education. Ultimately it will be detrimental to the patient care that is delivered by the graduates of our programs.

The need for the development and continuous quality improvement of the nurse educator workforce is not confined to the novice educator. We must consider what professional development models are most effective in supporting ongoing development of faculty at any career stage, to ensure continued engagement and relevance in the role. Some recent reports call for a radical transformation of the educational system in which nursing students are prepared to keep pace with the transforming health care system. The recommendations in these reports envision a role for the professoriate that is systems oriented, integrated into the practice environment, interprofessional in nature, and characterized by partnerships and collaborations.

For example, recommendations released from the proceedings of the 2017 Macy Foundation Conference regarding time-variable, competency-based health professions education call for (1) system redesign of faculty development, curricula, and learning environments; (2) creation of a learning continuum that encompasses education, training, and practice; (3) strengthened assessment efforts that demonstrate education and health care outcome linkages; (4) enhanced use of technology to support competency-based learning environments delivered using time-variable methods; and (5) effective models of outcome evaluation that measure educational outcomes linked to health care outcomes (Josiah Macy Jr. Foundation, 2017). Implementing these recommendations will require academic leaders to reconceptualize the nurse educator role as one that exists within a continuum of education-practice environments, cultivating interprofessional partnerships to design, implement, and evaluate relevant curricula.

Similarly, the AACN released the 2016 report *Advancing Healthcare Transformation: A New Era for Academic Nursing,* which focused on schools of nursing situated within academic health centers (AHCs) and the role they play in partnership with practice in transforming health care. The report called for the full integration of academic nursing into the AHC practice setting including participation in governance and care delivery, development of nurse leaders within the system, expansion of interprofessional research programs in partnership with other health profession schools, development of collaborative workforce plans, and integration into the AHCs' population health initiatives. For nurse educators to engage as full partners in these activities requires them to have, at a minimum, expertise in systems thinking, knowledge of emerging health care models, and skill in leadership, negotiations, collaboration, and advocacy.

Creating learning environments that facilitate the achievement of desired student learning outcomes is an important responsibility of educators. But even more important, as a profession, do we have agreement on what the desired student learning outcomes should be across all types of nursing programs? Beyond the commonly cited student outcomes related to graduation rates, licensure, certification, and employment rates, it becomes difficult to identify widely adopted consistencies in the desired student learning outcomes across the curricula of our nursing programs.

Curriculum development can become an overwhelming endeavor for many faculty, and it is even more so without clarity regarding student learning outcomes. What is lacking among many educators is an understanding of how best to integrate professional standards and concepts into a curriculum in a coherent manner that does not overwhelm both educators and learners. Faculty too frequently begin curriculum development efforts by starting from "scratch," expending much time and energy. There is a preponderance of professional standards and guidelines for faculty to consider for inclusion in the curriculum, and the introduction of concept-based curricula has further added to the intricacy of curriculum development and program evaluation. While this is not an attempt to advocate for a standardized national curriculum, it is a call for identifying strategies to ensure that graduates emerge from all of our programs with the consistent set of skills they need to deliver quality care. Having such conversations among interdisciplinary education and practice partners at local, regional, or national levels would help faculty develop relevant curricula connected to patient care outcomes and require students to consistently connect their learning to improving patient outcomes across all levels of practice.

Developing skill in outcome evaluation is a nurse educator competency that has not received a lot of attention in the literature to date. Given the increased focus on measuring and evaluating the achievement of student learning outcomes, not only in nursing education, but also in higher education and by accrediting bodies and other interested stakeholders (e.g., funding agencies, legislative bodies), the future quality of our nursing education programs would be well served by nurse educators who are skilled in designing outcome evaluation strategies. It is also important to demonstrate competence with methodologies that lead to the valid and reliable measurement of student learning outcomes. Learning how to most effectively measure student learning outcomes across the academic continuum is a future priority for nurse educators.

Historically, nursing education has had a tendency to address the needs of students and faculty in undergraduate and graduate programs separately and discretely, with graduate nursing education receiving less attention in the research literature. As a result, rather than viewing the educational process as a continuum across the academic spectrum, an artificial separation of undergraduate and graduate education has been created in the literature. With the increased emphasis on designing programs that promote academic progression and move learners more quickly across undergraduate/graduate program boundaries (e.g., RN to MSN; BSN to PhD or DNP), future directions for the nurse educator role include nurse educators gaining an understanding of how best to facilitate learner development as the learner progresses from entry-level nursing practice to advanced nursing practice.

With the design of new academic progression models typically achieved in compressed time frames, it is important for nurse educators not to lose sight of the professional socialization of learners when creating learning experiences. Effective strategies for developing the professional identity and socialization of learners and measuring student learning outcomes related to these concepts remain somewhat elusive in the literature. In an attempt to address this question, the NLN (2010) developed a framework of outcomes and competencies with identified outcomes related to human flourishing, nursing judgment, professional identity, and spirit of inquiry that have been leveled across all program types, demonstrating a logical progression of learner development in these areas. An examination of the identified outcomes illustrates that they are foundational to the professional socialization and identity of all learners and are worthy of consideration by the nursing profession as a common set of professional socialization outcomes that, at a minimum, all nursing students can be expected to achieve.

The future role of the nurse educator in clinical learning environments is another area that deserves serious reconsideration. Our clinical education models remain largely unchanged despite repeated national calls for transforming them to better reflect emerging health care delivery systems. We need to consider the focus of the learning experiences in the clinical education models in use in our nursing programs. Are the learning experiences designed to develop the student's clinical decision-making skills, or is the focus more on "doing" psychomotor nursing skills and administering medications a prescribed number of times so the learner can be "checked off" on the given skill? Becoming proficient in the safe performance of nursing skills is important; however, there is a danger in focusing on the acquisition of skills and not providing students with opportunities to engage in patient care situations that require the application of clinical judgment and an evaluation of patient outcomes. Imbedding the performance of nursing skills within the context of clinical decisions that impact patient outcomes is a priority.

The dramatic changes happening in the clinical environment demand unflinching attention to patient outcomes. This, in turn, requires nurse educators to design clinical learning experiences that directly link learning outcomes to clinical decision-making that has an impact on patient care outcomes. For the design of future clinical education models, nurse educators must embrace the notion of radical change in clinical education to produce competent graduates. Clinical models such as dedicated education units (DEUs) have demonstrated the potential to positively affect student learning. Are there other clinical immersion models to be considered that can facilitate the acquisition of clinical decision-making skills? What are the characteristics of a clinical learning environment that successfully fosters professional development of students? How do we measure growth in clinical decision-making as a student learning outcome?

Nurse educators need to be skilled in creating clinical "learning communities" that allow students to flourish in the environment, in contrast to the fragmented system of clinical experiences that many students currently encounter. Such change cannot be achieved without the collaboration and cooperation of practice partners. Intentionally cultivating the learning community triad of student-teacher-practicing nurse is an essential element to the success of any clinical model that is designed to effectively transition the learner from the educational environment to the practice environment.

The nurse educator role of the future will continue to be significantly impacted by the use of technology in the clinical setting and in the classroom. The use of instructional technology has historically been the primary focus of the nursing education literature. This focus needs to expand to include the use of technology in supporting the assessment and evaluation of student learning outcomes and understanding the evolving application of technology in learning analytics. Furthermore, nurse educators need to increase their competence with the use of technology in the clinical setting. Electronic health records, technology-supported clinical decision-making, and telehealth all have major implications for nursing practice and will require nurse educators to incorporate these concepts into student learning experiences.

SUMMARY

The scholarly work that is contained within the pages of this book demonstrates the influence that the NLN Core Competencies of Nurse Educators has had on the role of the nurse educator over the past 13 years. This work also points toward the future, with the core competencies continuing to provide a framework for individuals in their practice as nurse educators, researchers who are searching for the next research question, students who are exploring what it means to embrace nursing education as a career, and faculty who are designing curricula to prepare the next generation of nurse educators. Since their initial publication in 2005, it is clear that the NLN Core Competencies for Nurse Educators have influenced a greater understanding of the many aspects of the nurse educator role. They remain a relevant model to guide the future development of the nurse educator role and influence the quality of nursing education.

References

American Association of Colleges of Nursing. (2016). *Advancing healthcare transformation: A new era for academic nursing.* Washington, DC: Author. Retrieved from http://www.aacnnursing.org/Portals/42/Publications/AACN-New-Era-Report.pdf

American Association of Colleges of Nursing. (2018, March 26). *Defining scholarship for academic nursing task force consensus position statement.* Washington, DC: Author. Retrieved from http://www.aacnnursing.org/Portals/42/News/Position-Statements/Defining-Scholarship.pdf

Halstead, J. A. (2007). *Nurse educator competencies: Creating an evidence-based practice for nurse educators.* New York, NY: National League for Nursing.

Josiah Macy Jr. Foundation. (2017). *Achieving competency-based, time-variable, health professions education: Recommendations from the Macy Foundation Conference.* Retrieved from http://macyfoundation.org/docs/macy_pubs/JMF_CBTVHPE_Summary_web_JMF.pdf

National League for Nursing. (2010). *Outcomes and competencies for graduates of practical/vocational, diploma, associate degree, baccalaureate, master's, practice doctorate, and research doctorate programs in nursing.* New York, NY: Author.

Valiga, T. (2007). Creating an evidence-based practice for nurse educators. In J. A. Halstead (Ed.), *Nurse educator competencies: Creating an evidence-based practice for nurse educators* (pp. 169–174). New York, NY: National League for Nursing.